The Heartmates® Journal

D1245192

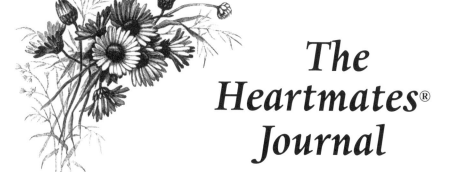

The Heartmates® Journal

A Companion for Partners of People with Serious Illness

Second edition

Rachael Freed

Fairview Press
Minneapolis

Fairview Press is a division of Fairview Health Services, a community-focused health system affiliated with the University of Minnesota and providing a complete range of services, from the prevention of illness and injury to care for the most complex medical conditions. For a free current catalog of Fairview Press titles, please call toll-free 1-800-544-8207. Or visit our Web site at www.fairviewpress.org.

First edition: 1995 MinervaPress
Second edition: 2002 Fairview Press

ISBN: 1-57749-122-X

Printed in Canada
06 05 04 03 02   6 5 4 3 2 1

Interior by Dorie McClelland, Spring Book Design
Cover by Laurie Ingram Design (www.laurieingramdesign.com)
Cover image from an original painting by Igor Levashov, courtesy Winters Fine
        Art, Carmel, California

Grateful acknowledgment is made for permission to quote from *Mainstay* © 1988 by Maggie Strong (Little, Brown & Co.) and *Fear of Fifty* © 1994 by Erica Jong (HarperCollins).

Disclaimer
This publication is designed to provide accurate and authoritative information in regard to the subject matter covered. It is sold with the understanding that the publisher is not engaged in the provision or practice of medical, nursing, or professional healthcare advice or services in any jurisdiction. If medical advice or other professional assistance is required, the services of a qualified and competent professional should be sought. Fairview Press is not responsible or liable, directly or indirectly, for any form of damages whatsoever resulting from the use (or misuse) of information contained in or implied by these documents.

Strange is our situation here on earth.
Each of us comes for a short visit, not knowing why,
    yet sometimes seeming to divine a purpose.
From the standpoint of daily life, however,
    there is one thing we do know:
    that we are here for the sake of others;
    above all, for those on whose smile and well-being
    our own happiness depends;
    and also for the countless unknown souls with whose fate
    we are connected by a bond of sympathy.
Many times a day I realize how much my outer and inner life
    is built upon the labor of others,
    both living and dead, and how earnestly I must exert myself
    in order to give in return
    as much as I have received and am still receiving.

Albert Einstein

CONTENTS

FOREWORD

I feel privileged to write this foreword for a book I find immeasurably helpful, and for an author who is a dear friend. First, the author. Rachael and I have collaborated in some capacity for each of the past five decades. We became acquainted in the 1960s, when she was my high school English teacher (she cringes when I reveal this fact). She had a small class of sixteen students in the advanced-placement English program. My friends and I found her amazingly challenging, fun, idealistic, "cool," and extremely demanding. A few months ago, we had a thirty-five-year high school reunion, and many present gave Rachael credit for their success in various fields, all of which require a command of language.

In the 1970s, Rachael and I worked together again, this time to create the Program Concerned with Death and Dying at Mt. Sinai Hospital in Minneapolis. It was a forerunner to hospice and to bioethics committees. Rachael's great vision led us to cutting-edge caregiving at a time when death was unspeakable.

In the 1980s, Rachael wrote the book *Heartmates,* and we traveled together to several U.S. cities to teach cardiology centers the art of caring for spouses and families. Her personal experience, bolstered by her professional experience, created an engaging speaker who touched the hearts of the audience, both professional and lay.

In the 1990s, we collaborated on the writing of my book, *Finding Your Way: Families and the Cancer Experience.* Rachael cheered me on. Of course, there is nothing more exciting for an old English teacher than to see one of her students succeed in the world of writing!

It is now the decade of the 2000s. We are again touching each other's lives in her creation of this exceptional book, *The Heartmates Journal.* If you have stayed with me during my nostalgic walk through the past, I now want to address the quality and value of this book.

As a psychologist who works primarily with people and their families who are dealing with serious chronic illness, I can attest to the value of writing as a tool for emotional healing. Studies have verified this, but even without the studies the anecdotal evidence is overwhelming.

Writing is a release; writing is a healer. Whether the disease is heart disease, cancer, multiple sclerosis, arthritis, COPD, or a myriad of other chronic illnesses, the dynamics are very similar. One must grieve losses; one must create a new "normal." The old lifestyle is a casualty in the move toward acceptance, not only for the person with the disease but also for the loved ones.

Too often the focus of healthcare professionals and friends and family is solely on the person with the illness. The partner, children, parents, and siblings are not recognized as hurting. This book acknowledges the needs of those walking the pathway with the sick one, revealing their very real struggle to find balance between self-care and other-care. Rachael skillfully addresses many of the hidden reactions of the caregiver ("heartmate") and encourages the expression of emotions. She urges an optimistic approach to coping by naming and developing qualities that will contribute to good mental health.

One of the greatest gifts offered by this book is the gift of normalcy. It allows the heartmate to repeatedly confront the fact that, although many reactions may feel crazy, most are quite normal. The range of normal at a time of crisis is very broad. There is no one right way to react. Although there are threads of similarity in reactions of heartmates, no two people respond in quite the same way. Thus, Rachael's journal pages cover a broad range of possible experiences and suggest a variety of related topics to think and write about.

I strongly urge you to take the time to write. In the busiest time of your life, it is a lot to ask, but the rewards will be immeasurable. Your life and the life of your partner, child, or whoever surrounds you will be affected. Take those feelings and ideas that are swimming around in your head and put them down in black and white. You won't regret it. And your old high school English teacher would be so proud!

Wishing you inspired writing and emotional healing,

Gail A. Noller, PsyD, licensed psychologist
and author of *Finding Your Way: Families
and the Cancer Experience*

A WORD FROM THE AUTHOR

Hope is the thing with feathers
That perches in the soul
And sings the tune without the words
And never stops at all.

Emily Dickinson

This book is dedicated to caregiving partners. No matter which illness, diagnosis, or crisis event your loved one has experienced, in that moment, your life changed forever. You became a heartmate, though others may call you by another name: informal caregiver, family caregiver, well spouse.

Your life became inextricably bound to a situation not personally yours or of your making. Your identity—like your feelings, hopes, and dreams—became invisible, went underground. Your needs became secondary to the needs of your partner.

Though your mate may be the most beloved in your life, this is the truth: you share a common path, but you each have your own journey. Out of love, guilt, sadness, obligation, or fear, you may have tried to go on your loved one's journey. But your partner's journey—what is happening to and inside him or her—is different than your own.

Once the realization is accepted
that even between the closest human beings infinite distances
continue to exist,
a wonderful living side by side can grow up,
if they succeed in loving the distance between them
which makes it possible for each to see the other whole
against the sky.

Rainer Maria Rilke, Letters 1929

This book was designed to assist you in a most significant spiritual task: to lead you back to yourself so you can reclaim and respect your journey. I hope it will be a source of healing tears, healing laughter, wholeness—and peace.

To every heartmate using this journal, believe in the hope and possibility of recovery. May your healing be complete.

Rachael Freed
Minneapolis, Minnesota
2002

ACKNOWLEDGMENTS

I am grateful to so many for their support and cooperation in making this book possible. In particular, I want to acknowledge those heart-mates who have contributed to the healing of others by appearing in the video series, *Portrait of the Heartmate,* and for permitting their heartfelt thoughts to appear here: Sharon Anstett, Dorothy Atkinson, Bonnie Barland, Shussie Blumenthal, Mary Charpentier, Ethelyn Cohen, Mitzi Crowley, Ruth Fram, Lavonne Garcia, Yleen Joselyn, Robin Lalor-Schleck, Gretchen Mahigan, Cynthia L. McCurtain, and Ardis Niemann Noonan.

I am grateful beyond words for discovering the values and princi-ples of journal writing, Al-Anon, and Reform Judaism, which guide my spiritual development; for the nurture of belonging in those com-munities; and for the love of family and friends, who continue to support me on my journey.

INTRODUCTION

Illness is a tear in the fabric of family life. The entire family is wounded by, and thus suffers from, one family member's serious illness. Since the illness can't be undone, the family must reweave the fabric so it is once again whole, though it will be different than before. The goal is healing. The whole tapestry of family health and human feelings must be addressed, not just the part that shows the damage.

Studies indicate that social support is essential to a full recovery for both patients and their heartmates. When they return home after hospitalization, they are on their own, often isolated from others who share their concerns. Many live far from the hospital where diagnosis and treatment were given. They cannot participate in outpatient educational and support programs.

Heartmates' recoveries are complicated by the fact that the physical illness is not theirs, but a loved one's. Most heartmates, busy attending to their patient's needs, don't even realize that they, too, have been wounded. Without self-reflection or prompting from someone who understands, heartmates never even consider the possibility that they also need to recover.

Society eagerly but erroneously believes that family life returns to normal when the patient survives. My personal experience was different from everyone's expectation: my family was not untouched and did not bounce back. I didn't know what to do, what was expected of me, so I did what many women do in a crisis. I jumped right into my Superwoman suit and tried to handle everything! I felt responsible for keeping him alive. And then it was on to recovery and more unknowns.

I came to realize that we, partners of the patients, are also in recovery. We have been so busy caring for our mates that we haven't paid enough attention to our own needs. We have to find the right balance between caring for them and for ourselves so that all of us can recover as fully as possible.

The Heartmates Journal: A Companion for Partners of People with Serious Illness helps combat the isolation and lack of support that so often hamper long-term recovery. It invites heartmates to participate in their own recovery, to learn how to help themselves heal by reading, journal writing, and meditating. Weekly exercises provide practical techniques to support heartmates coping with the ongoing changes in their lives due to their partner's illness.

Most caregivers are women. Society has trained women to take care of their men and their children, but not themselves. And men, too, sometimes neglect themselves for the sake of their loved ones. For these reasons, self-care is a top priority of this journal.

Some people may know to take care of themselves through diet and exercise. Others may have a trusted friend or a competent counselor to talk with. And still others may be comforted by their religious faith. But most women—and many men—lack even basic education about the importance of self-care. Fewer still are trained in the attitudes and practices of self-care.

Heartmates are vicarious victims of trauma. For them, self-care is not a luxury. It is a necessity. If they are going to recover and grow while simultaneously caregiving for their mate and supporting their family, heartmates need to heal their body, feelings, mind, and spirit. It is just as necessary to address their needs for privacy and quiet as for social connection, support, stimulation, meaning, and service.

Ruth Fram, an experienced heartmate, wrote about her recovery:

> I have had many years of coping with the traumas of life. I'm made of "tough stuff." I have learned to be more philosophical about life, to I take one day at a time and cherish that day. I am happy to report that I still have the ability to laugh and I make sure that some laughter is part of my day. . . . Even though I take my responsibilities very seriously, I am not a martyr. I am the caregiver and perhaps I don't get out socially as much as I might want to, but I keep a part of me for just me. If I give all of me, I can be destroyed as an individual and then have nothing to give. I am sixty-seven years old and still learning. . . . Everyone should have another interest that they are passionate about. For me it is needlework.

The Heartmates Journal was created to help heartmates heal so they can live fully and with great optimism and wisdom, like Ruth.

One purpose of this journal is to comfort and support heartmates who feel alone or frozen in place by fear. Once they are liberated from the deep freeze, heartmates can take advantage of the positive opportunities in the health crisis. They will discover that it's okay to feel again and return to the rest of the world.

Another purpose is to challenge heartmates to accept where they are—a basic step in furthering growth. I don't believe we are given illness in order to grow, but I do believe that once we are touched by a life-threatening illness, there is a natural opportunity to grow and to question much of what we have taken for granted. Your own experience will evoke questions about priorities, values, the meaning of life (particularly your life), your spiritual purpose, and God or your higher power.

How to Use This Journal

The Heartmates Journal is designed for your personal use as an interactive, year-long recovery resource. The body of the book is organized by week rather than by day. Daily entries are too overwhelming, too much to take on, when you are grieving and healing. The book follows the course of a year, but you will have your own calendar of recovery that won't necessarily begin in January and end in December.

You'll find a balance of messages, thoughts, and information as well as space to record your recovery. Each week offers a quotation followed by a short discussion, an affirmation, suggestions for thinking and writing, and three "qualities"—desirable characteristics—to meditate on. The entries are short and to the point, because heartmates, particularly in the early months of grieving, may experience difficulty concentrating for any length of time.

I have tried to provide guidance that is both general enough to mean something to all heartmates, and specific enough to apply to your personal circumstances. If you would like to choose a different focus for any given week, you will find additional quotations in appendix B. You may find them more meaningful than those provided in the body of this book, or you can use them as additional reading anytime during your recovery and beyond. In addition, all the affirmations appear in appendix C. You may want to mark those that are especially important to you.

The personal "qualities" for meditation are meant to relate to the focus of the week and are appropriate to a particular phase of recovery; however, you may occasionally wish to replace suggested qualities with others that might be more appropriate to your experience. A complete list of qualities is given in appendix D.

The three parts of this journal are organized to correspond to the progression of recovery:

Part I: Early Recovery: "Help, I Don't Get It!" (the first twenty weeks)
Part II: Midrecovery: "The Long Haul" (the next twenty weeks)
Part III: Toward Full Recovery: "I Can See the Light" (the final twelve weeks)

Each part touches on self-care; feelings; isolation and support; meaning and values; spiritual issues; and relationship "re-pair," including physical intimacy, partnership, and family concerns.

When a topic is revisited in a later part of the journal, the focus goes deeper. Early months stress recognition and acknowledgment of your new reality; middle months focus on acceptance of this reality; later months aid integration and encourage celebration.

At the end of the book are pages for writing down specific concerns. Writing notes there will help you remember all the things you are responsible for during your partner's recovery: important phone numbers, prescriptions, questions for the doctors, special recipes, personal notes.

The Chaotic Course of Healing

Although the book is divided into three parts corresponding to three distinct phases, I warn you, there is no straight path to healing. Each of us, unique and beautiful, must chart and follow his or her own course. So, although part I, a twenty-week section, focuses on issues that occur mainly in the acute months of the recovery process, you may find you want to return to part I and tend to some of those issues even as you near the end of the book.

If I could predict an orderly, straightforward recovery for heart-mates, I would. I know from my own experience and that of other heartmates, however, that chaos reigns. Don't let the linear structure of this book discourage you. Instead, use it as a means for setting some order to the chaos you are experiencing.

You may choose to read along until you come upon an entry that fits your immediate need, then write and meditate about it. Certain topics may interest you for only a few days, while you may choose to write about others for a month or even longer. Some people open books randomly, believing that what they open to is what they need. Please use the journal in a way that is right for you.

Note that the journal weeks are not yet dated. I understand that each heartmate's healing journey is unique. I encourage you to date the journal sequence according to your recovery in a way that suits you.

Two integral components of recovery are celebration and humor. You are invited to remember their importance in your entries throughout the year. Laughter can be as healing as tears. Each achievement, each sign of progress in your recovery journey, is an occasion for celebration.

CELEBRATION

Ours is a culture that stresses speed and efficiency and has little patience for mourning or the lengthy healing process. We therefore have few rituals to celebrate healing. When progress is made, goals are met, and anniversaries are marked, these special moments deserve to be celebrated.

The recommended reading list (appendix A) includes books about ritual, although none specifically apply to celebrating your family's healing. Talk with each other about celebrations that suit you. Design your own individual, couple, and family celebrations. Enjoy them as often as you can.

HUMOR

A great contributor to the healing process, humor—playfulness—allows us to see with refreshing clarity. Humor can aid your recovery; revel in it whenever possible. It lightens the weight of your burden and puts your situation in perspective. Laughter may indeed be the best medicine, as therapeutic as tears.

JOURNAL WRITING

Some heartmates lack a confidante to share their pain and joy. Others prize their privacy. Still others find it difficult or impossible to share with a friend or a group. For many people, then, writing is the ideal medium of expression.

Using the weekly exercises as a springboard, take a few minutes daily or a couple times a week to write in the journal. In doing so, you will be demonstrating self-care. You'll be caring enough about yourself to make time to think and write about your concerns.

You will find suggestions each week to stimulate your thinking and writing. You may have a different response to a quotation than my comments present, or the reading may evoke a deep, personal memory that you prefer to write about. Remember, the suggestions are just that—suggestions.

Journal writing aids your healing by facilitating storytelling. In order to heal from any crisis situation, you need to tell your story. Telling and retelling your story helps you understand, accept, and finally integrate the health crisis experience, as well as your emotional, mental, and spiritual reactions to it. If you don't have a willing ear to listen to you, or you feel more comfortable with privacy, the journal is a perfect place to tell your story. You can change your mind or your story without having to make yourself understood to someone else. You can repeat as much as you need. You can go back to earlier writing to trace your path and progress.

Expressing emotions is an essential task in the healing process. Writing in your journal is a safe way to air your feelings. It is also a method to explore and uncover feelings that may be otherwise inaccessible. What you may not feel free to say aloud to someone can be safely articulated in your journal, lifting those feelings out of the dark and bringing them to light. Via pen on paper, you can discover and vent.

Letting go of the old and accepting the new is another important component of healing. Parts of your personality will struggle with what has happened. Those parts prefer to yearn for the past, rather than surrender to what's happened and move into the present. Putting words on paper can help you to accept reality.

When you write about your daily activities, feelings, and thoughts, you can begin to make sense of changes in your life. Rereading old journal entries can help you track the development and existence of behavioral patterns that you might not otherwise notice. Writing about these patterns may increase your understanding, giving you the impetus to let go of outdated habits and establish new ones.

Maybe the most important activity in the healing process is searching for meaning. Writing in a journal creates a stable record of your progress. A crisis makes you vulnerable, and this vulnerability is not something to be feared or despised. It offers you an opportunity for great inner growth and spiritual healing. Journaling will give you regular, undisturbed quiet time to pursue your thoughts, your feelings, your questions, and your concerns. Writing provides you a way to actively participate in and chronicle your journey.

If you maintain an open attitude as you write, you may experience insights, inner guidance, and fuller understanding. Insights often come in a flash and, like dreams, are quickly forgotten. Write down your flashes of insight in your journal. You can always think and write about the meaning of the insight at a later time.

Find a special place for writing in your journal. Make it a cozy and comfortable place, a place away from the distractions of everyday life, such as the phone and television. If you can schedule it daily, or every other day, you will find it easier to build the habit of regular journal writing. Carry your journal with you and write in the doctor's waiting room, on a park bench, while caring for your napping grandchildren, or whenever you have a "found" moment. (I like to carry a small notebook with me so I can jot down flashes of insight, ideas, and so on. Later I incorporate these notes into my journal writing.)

There is no one right way to use this journal. During the first few weeks, you will probably devise your own writing schedule and style. Some heartmates, for example, like to journal in the early morning or late at night when everyone else is asleep. Others like to take breaks throughout the day to write in their journals.

It's okay to be creative. Creativity is helpful in healing. Experiment with style, and feel free to change your writing to express who you are and how you feel. Some people print, others write in cursive. Some keep neat journals, while other journals are barely legible.

Heartmate Cynthia L. McCurtain wrote this poem in her journal during one of her husband's hospitalizations:

the pain comes and washes over me
i walk out in the hall so that you won't see
i leave tears on the walls
on the floors in a private corner
and breathe deeply
come back and smile.
it's not so hard to bring you smiles
for you are my happiness
my heart holds your ache
and your anger
it belongs to me too.
i could tear down a wall with my bare hands right now
but i won't and i don't
i'll just sit quietly for you now
for you always.

i can't change things
i just pray for the courage to accept things the way they are
and my courage comes.
you have always been my strength
let me be yours.
let us be each other's—always.

MEDITATION

When you hear the word "meditation," you may imagine a lone monk at the top of a high mountain or someone sitting silently in the lotus position for long hours. But meditation is simply a mental action—a conscious, deliberate use of thought for a specific purpose.

Meditation is a practical and purposeful discipline, like regular physical exercise. As physical exercise fosters rehabilitation by tuning and strengthening the body, so meditation aids recovery by tuning and using the mind in a purposeful way. You can use meditation to build or maintain an idea or energize a desirable quality, such as compassion.

As you train your mind to be focused, orderly, reflective, quiet, attentive, open, and receptive, these characteristics will carry into your everyday and spiritual life. You'll find that meditation will increase your awareness of the energies you need in your daily recovery. It can quiet and calm your mind, establishing a stable foundation for decision making. It can help you cope with and grow from the health crisis. And, when you focus your mind on questions of identity, meaning, and purpose, it can help you approach your real self, deepening your spirituality.

HOW TO MEDITATE

Meditation is a discipline requiring patience and repetition. Before you make a long-term commitment, experiment with the meditation techniques described in the following pages. If you decide to continue, be kind to yourself. Know that your expectations may not immediately correspond to the reality of your practice.

You may choose to meditate daily or two or three times a week. Remember, acquiring any new habit is a challenge. Inertia, lethargy, and the old excuses of not having the time or being too busy will be tough to overcome. Your reluctance may get stronger before you overcome it, but perseverance and commitment will yield marvelous results and will enhance your healing process.

Because meditating on qualities may be an entirely new concept, here is a detailed description of the process. You can follow these instructions until you're ready to adapt the discipline to suit yourself.

Phase 1: Preparation

Sit comfortably in a quiet place, away from distractions, where you can have privacy for ten to twenty minutes. Reread the weekly exercise. Choose a quality—such as detachment, gratitude, or joy—listed at the bottom of the page. You might select one that is most inviting or familiar, or choose a quality that you think you altogether lack. If none of the qualities listed in the weekly exercise fits your needs, look through appendix D and select one that corresponds to your present circumstances.

Close your eyes (if it will help you focus inward and avoid being visually distracted) and take a few deep breaths. Relax your body as much as you can, keeping your spine straight and your feet in contact with the floor. Take a few more deep breaths and focus on your breathing to help calm your feelings and empty your mind. Your goal is to be relaxed but not passive, tension-free but alert, with your full attention on the quality chosen for meditation. Bring the quality into your mind with each breath.

Phase 2: Reflection

During this phase of the meditation, you will think about your chosen personal quality and its many aspects. You may want to follow all the suggestions in this section, or focus on only one or two.

For the next three to five minutes, think about your chosen personal quality. Imagine the quality written inside your mind. Imagine it as written in an appropriate color and lettering. Think of words, phrases, or ideas that you normally associate with this quality. Think of synonyms for the quality; think of opposites. Think of how you feel about this quality in yourself and in others. Identify people who have this quality. Think about situations when you've needed this quality. Think about times when you have used it and how it affected you and the situation. Think about how your recovery or your family's would be different if you had more of this quality available. Think about how it affects your life, your family's life, life in the broader world. Think about questions you may have about this quality: its source, how scarce or abundant it is, what stops its spread throughout the world, what advantageous effect this quality might have in your personal life and in the world.

When you have thought about the quality as fully as you can, return your attention to your breathing and take a few deep breaths.

Phase 3: Reception

This phase of meditation goes beyond reflection. Your goal is to hold your mind open, alert, and receptive, inviting the unconscious mind to join the conscious mind so you can receive deeper understanding or insight. Continue to sit comfortably and focus on your breathing. It is not necessary to change your breathing pattern; just observe it as a way of focusing inward.

Now gather all your ideas, thoughts, and feelings about the quality and imagine placing them into a clear, crystal bowl. Hold the bowl up and imagine the rays of the sun shining into your bowl of reflections. Now focus your attention on the bowl and its contents. Notice any thoughts or feelings you have as you hold the bowl.

Stay expectant for one to two minutes or as long as you can remain focused. Entertain any changes that happen as you observe the bowl, its contents, and the sun's rays. If there is no response, acknowledge your disappointment and the difficulty of maintaining patience and receptivity. Awareness, insight, and understanding don't always happen right away, especially if you are new to meditation. The opportunity will present itself again when you next meditate. Because meditation is a way of opening yourself, insights also may come to you between this meditation and your next.

Phase 4: Transforming Vision into Action

This final phase is also called "creative meditation." It combines the information and energy from the reflective and receptive phases, using your mind and imagination to bring your awareness into action. Transforming awareness so that its energy can be used in the world is the essence of the mind-body connection. It makes awareness practical and purposeful, helping you cope with the daily struggles and adaptations of living with your mate's illness. Spend no more than three to five minutes on this last phase of the meditation.

Focus again on your breathing as a technique of holding your attention on the quality. Sit comfortably, and again collect your thoughts, feelings, and insights. Now, think about a current situation in your life in which having this quality would be beneficial. Imagine that just before you enter into the situation, you call on the energy of the quality to be with you. Then imagine yourself entering the scene and expressing the new energy as you live the event. Notice how you feel different, how your actions are different, how your view of yourself and the situation changes when you have that energy.

If you choose, you can now take the time to imagine other scenes that you need to cope with in your life: at home, with your mate, at work, with friends. Notice the effect of the quality on these situations—for better or worse.

Before you leave your comfortable chair, take a few more breaths and clear your mind and feelings. You may want to write notes in your journal before you return to your daily routine. Remember, too, that you may find it useful to meditate more than once on the same quality. Stay with it as long as you continue to strengthen your understanding of the quality or benefit from the focus.

Variations

Continuously motivating yourself to make the changes that you've written about in your journal can be a challenge. In order to make these changes a real part of your recovery, you will need to keep thinking about them until they become second nature. For each weekly exercise, repeat the affirmation and visualize your chosen quality throughout the day, not just when you're writing in your journal.

Write each week's quality on a three-by-five card, using large letters and appropriate colors. Add embellishments to the card to attract the energy of the quality. Put the card in a place where you will notice it. My favorite places, for example, are the refrigerator door and the bathroom mirror. Look at the word often to keep its image present in your mind, even when you aren't paying full conscious attention to it.

Imagine how you can express the quality in your recovery. Watch how others in your life express this quality. Write in your journal about the quality and your observations of how it is affecting your life.

When you stop noticing the card, it may be time to give the quality new life by creating a new card with a different design or moving the card to another conspicuous location. Not noticing the card can also signal that it's time to move on to a new quality. You may want to post a card with a new quality each week as you move to the next exercise in your journal. Or you may decide to focus on a quality for a month or longer, depending on the effect the quality is having in your recovery. On the other hand, don't be afraid to change qualities. You can always come back to a quality later.

Another possibility is to focus on the affirmation in the weekly exercise. Write the affirmation on a three-by-five card, and put it where you will see it. Each time you see it, read it aloud to yourself (facing a mirror, if possible). Even if you don't believe you can live the affirmation, given how you feel or where you are in your recovery, repeat it aloud to yourself in an assured voice. Repetition of the affirmation will increase the possibility that you can live it and experience its positive energy. In the meantime, try "acting as if" it is true for you.

MENTAL IMAGERY

In the adult world, mental images are rarely discussed or taken seriously. They are considered to be the products of children's imaginations, the senility of the aged, or the delusions of the mentally ill. Imagery doesn't get the respect it deserves in our culture, even though in some arenas—like athletic training, self-esteem enhancement, and cancer treatment—imagery is consciously used as a resource.

The imagination is a sophisticated human function that integrates components of the mind and the feelings. Beneath our conscious awareness, our mind and emotions form our interpretations of reality.

These images are the basis of our world view and the foundation of our actions. We trust our images; they influence what we think and do. We respond to our images as if they were reality.

When we are unaware of what our images are, we are controlled by them. If your image of the hospital is a place with a competent and caring staff, for example, you're prone to be satisfied with the quality of care your partner receives. If you see the hospital as a place of helplessness and isolation, you will have a tendency to view it as an impersonal, untrustworthy place. The truth is somewhere in-between these two examples, but it's the images that form your reality.

Until this health crisis, you probably trusted your images: the security of your lifestyle, your relationship with your mate, your expectations for your future. The wound of your partner's illness shattered these images of reality. Part of your process of healing is to repair them.

The process of repairing your images includes becoming aware of those that no longer match reality. You need to grieve the loss of these images before you can build new ones that mirror your present circumstances. Letting go of obsolete images will help you live with the new reality that includes your partner's illness.

My husband's heart attack, for example, changed my image of who he really was. I had never given much thought to his mortality. In the life-threatening crisis that brought him to a bed in the coronary care unit, I understood what I had not noticed or thought about before. He was mortal. This meant that he would die. Maybe not at that moment, but he wouldn't live forever.

The thought came as a great surprise. I knew that I would die; that realization had come with my mother's death ten years earlier. But I had never applied that knowledge to my husband. He was an invincible man; not only was he physically strong and active, his life energy had always seemed unfaltering.

That night in the cardiac care unit, the man I saw looking out at me from the tubes, wires, and machinery was a half-bald, gray-faced, middle-aged man. Where had my invulnerable hero gone? Who was this sick and aging man, his blue eyes flecked with fear and disbelief?

Why had I never noticed time passing? Why had I never brought the image of my mate up to date? My perception of him was unconnected to the real world, with its unrelenting passage of time.

As painful as it was to look time in the face, there was no way to avoid it. Little by little, reminded by my own graying hair and the lines in my face, I began to integrate a new image, making it more realistic and current. In time, my image of us as vital human beings became enriched with the maturity and wisdom that comes with experience.

Your images may need an overhaul, too. If you want to work more with your images, see appendix E for imagery exercises adapted from *Heartmates*. They include a relaxation exercise, a guide for examining images, the Evening Review exercise, and an Evening Review on Boundaries.

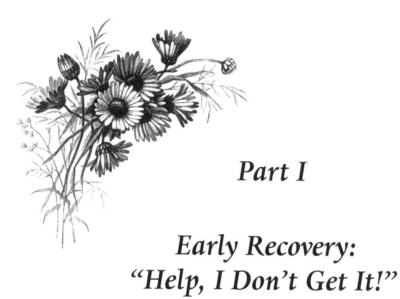

Part I

Early Recovery:
"Help, I Don't Get It!"

I remember telling the staff, even the doctors, "He can't come home yet: he's not ready, I'm not ready." I remember thinking, "How am I going to know if he's all right? Am I going to wake up and find out he's quit breathing? Would he get back okay every time he went for his walk?"

Mitzie, a heartmate

In the early weeks after a diagnosis, health crisis, or event, we sound as if we're experiencing the classic symptoms of shock. That's because we are in shock! Whether we are quiet or outgoing, organized or scattered, enthusiastic or detached, we are vicarious victims of trauma.

We experience our trauma in different ways. We may feel it in our bodies: we're stiff or we ache; we hold our jaws tight and we hunch our shoulders. We may be dizzy or shaky or nauseated. Our feelings toss us like we're riding bucking broncos: we're hopeful then depressed, grateful then resentful, relieved then scared, helpless then angry, even guilty. Our nearest, though not dearest, companion is anxiety. Our minds feel thick and slow, empty or scrambled. It's difficult to concentrate or remember.

Recognizing your shock, you need to take small steps to take care of yourself: Eat regularly and well; good nutrition is a must for recovery. Nap and rest frequently; make up for disrupted sleep. Walk daily; exercise is essential to maintain physical, mental, and emotional health. Take time to do things that you like to do by and for yourself.

Affirmation: I will be gentle and kind to myself today.

Related topics to think/write about:
1) List ways I can take care of myself each day. 2) Write my self-care activities into my daily schedule.

Qualities to meditate on: Calm–quiet–simplicity.

Date _____

This is the _____ _week of my recovery_ _____

_____
_____
_____
_____
_____
_____
_____
_____
_____
_____
_____
_____
_____
_____
_____
_____
_____
_____
_____
_____
_____
_____
_____
_____
_____
_____
_____
_____
_____

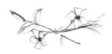

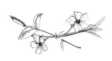

By letting go, it all gets done;
The world is won by those who let it go!
Tao Te Ching

The idea is to stop "doing" and assess what's needed. Then, use your energy for what really matters. If you just go, go, go because that's what you're used to doing, or you think that keeping busy will make this nightmare go away, you're fooling yourself.

Having your partner home from the hospital, no matter how well he or she is recovering, is exhausting as well as exhilarating. As a heartmate, you need to give yourself permission to let go of automatic routines. Your priority is to do only that which will directly take care of you and your recovering partner. Dishes and laundry will wait. If you're too uncomfortable leaving things undone, ask someone to help. Conserving energy for what's important is the key to making your way through the early days of recovery when so much is new and uncertain.

The idea of reorganizing your daily routine to accommodate a recovering partner is also fatiguing. As much as you can, incorporate coping skills that have worked in past crises. Your strengths are a base from which you can plan necessary change.

Affirmation: I will use my energy today to attend to what is truly important.

Related topics to think/write about:
1) List what I need to do daily during these first weeks of recovery for myself and my partner. Make another list of things that can wait. 2) Plan ways to replenish my energy.

Qualities to meditate on: Order–rest–surrender.

8

Date _____

This is the _____ *week of my recovery* _____

_____

_____

_____

_____

_____

_____

_____

_____

_____

_____

_____

_____

_____

_____

_____

_____

_____

_____

_____

_____

_____

_____

_____

_____

_____

_____

_____

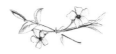

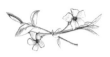

I was scared and I was tired, and I didn't talk to anyone who told me I should be.

Ethelyn, a heartmate

Heartmates tend to focus all their attention on the patient. We are deeply concerned about the welfare of our loved one whose life is threatened. Add sitting all day at the hospital, awaiting word from the doctor, being unaccustomed to the hospital's rules and regulations, trying to understand a strange technical language, and being removed from our familiar daily routines, it's no wonder heartmates are exhausted and anxious.

It is especially important that heartmates take good care of themselves. We, too, are experiencing a crisis from which we will need to heal and recover. By healing ourselves and maintaining our health, we will be better able to support our mate's recovery.

It is crucial that you balance your needs with your mate's needs. The old Buddhist wisdom, "Eat when you're hungry, drink when you're thirsty, sleep when you're tired," is sound advice for heartmates. Contemporary wisdom adds, "Get regular exercise, and ask others for support as you need it."

Affirmation: I accept the need to take care of myself.

Related topics to think/write about:
1) What kind of care do I need for my body, my feelings, my mind, my spirit? 2) How can I balance my needs, my partner's needs, my family's needs?

Qualities to meditate on: Balance–energy–renewal.

12

Date _____

This is the _____ *week of my recovery* _____

_____

_____

_____

_____

_____

_____

_____

_____

_____

_____

_____

_____

_____

_____

_____

_____

_____

_____

_____

_____

_____

_____

_____

_____

_____

_____

_____

_____

_____

_____

_____

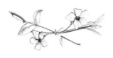

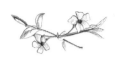

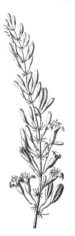

They were very good at the hospital with the education, the material they sent home with me, the meal plans. But then I had to execute the plans. I felt like I was a slave in the kitchen: meal planning took so much time; there were so many changes; I tried so hard to make meals to please him.

Gretchen, a heartmate

After years of meal planning and cooking, I was especially frightened to feel insecure and incompetent in the kitchen. Diet seemed to have life-and-death implications.

I thought I had to start over completely, learn to cook in a whole new way. If I didn't throw away everything in my freezer and count every milligram of salt and cholesterol, I believed my partner would keel over and die. I was so anxious. I tried to change everything all at once. I wish I had been guided with words like "gradual" and "moderation."

If you and your mate can talk about and plan dietary changes together, you both can implement a diet that is reasonable and manageable, and you can avoid becoming a nag or a culinary cop. Total deprivation of favorite foods will almost always backfire—a little planned "cheating" can go a long way! Remember:
- Lasting change is accomplished by building habits.
- Habits are formed over time and with practice.
- Take small enough steps to succeed.
- Share intermediate victories.
- Plan special treats to celebrate success.

Affirmation: I can change, a little bit every day.

Related topics to think/write about:
1) Make a list of lifestyle habits that I want to change.
2) Prioritize, breaking down each change into moderate, doable steps.

Qualities to meditate on: Celebration–creativity–patience.

16

Date _____

This is the _____ *week of my recovery* _____

_____
_____
_____
_____
_____
_____
_____
_____
_____
_____
_____
_____
_____
_____
_____
_____
_____
_____
_____
_____
_____
_____
_____
_____
_____
_____
_____
_____

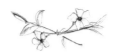

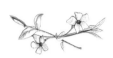

You probably have a slew of unspoken, unaddressed, and unanswered questions. They may torment you when you are trying to sleep or pop up at odd times, catching you unaware. You may find them circling around and around in your head.

Rachael Freed
Heartmates

As heartmates, we have questions and we want answers. But it isn't that simple. Medicine doesn't have all the answers, especially specific ones about your mate's progress and prognosis. Unaware of this fact or unwilling to accept it, you may think, "If I know, I'll feel less anxious." You have the right to ask questions, to seek information. At the same time, it is important to be realistic about answers you can expect.

Getting and understanding information is difficult for mates who are grieving and recovering from a crisis. Most of us realize that grief plays havoc with feelings. But few of us appreciate that our minds are also affected. Grievers have reduced ability to remember, concentrate, focus, organize ideas, make decisions.

I remember those early weeks of my recovery. A voracious reader since the first grade, I couldn't concentrate long enough to read a popular magazine. Worse, I had little patience with or humor about my limits.

Affirmation: I am entitled to have questions and answers.

Related topics to think/write about:
Write my list of questions, adding or checking off questions as appropriate and thinking about who can best provide answers.

Qualities to meditate on: Appreciation–comprehension–humor.

20

*Date*_____

*This is the_____week of my recovery*_____

_____
_____
_____
_____
_____
_____
_____
_____
_____
_____
_____
_____
_____
_____
_____
_____
_____
_____
_____
_____
_____
_____
_____
_____
_____
_____
_____
_____

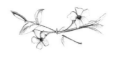

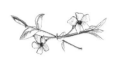

*Because people aren't mind readers, they aren't gonna know
you're feeling lousy if you don't tell them.*

Sharon, a heartmate

As difficult as it may be to ask for support, it is selfish and unwise
not to. Most heartmates are fortunate to have family and friends who
sincerely want to be supportive. They are kind and goodhearted, even
if they don't understand exactly what you are experiencing. If you
turn them away, you deprive them of the blessing of doing a good
deed for you. If you don't tell them what you need, they're left in
limbo, wanting to help but not knowing how.

An inner voice may tell you that you should handle the situation
yourself, you shouldn't be a bother to anyone, others have it worse, or
you're not deserving. Say no to that voice. It's wrong!

A health crisis is an extraordinary time in your life, your mate's life,
and your family's life. The manners, courtesy, and protocols you've
observed in ordinary situations just don't apply. Give others the
opportunity to give you the support you need, and receive that support as gracefully as you can.

Affirmation: I deserve support and I will ask for it.

Related topics to think/write about:
1) List things I need from others, from a hug to a hot meal.
2) Consider my feelings about giving to and receiving
from others.

Qualities to meditate on: Generosity–grace–openness.

Date _____

This is the _____ *week of my recovery* _____

_____

_____

_____

_____

_____

_____

_____

_____

_____

_____

_____

_____

_____

_____

_____

_____

_____

_____

_____

_____

_____

_____

_____

_____

_____

_____

_____

_____

_____

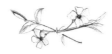

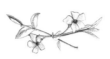

How would I support us? Where would we live? Who would
shovel the snow? Once I went through that, I was able to feel
inside that, "Gee, I hope to God this doesn't happen. I would be
very sad, but I would make it."

Robin, a heartmate

When my husband had a heart attack, our children were just thirteen and eleven. Prior to the event I had always been confident that with talent, hard work, and good luck we would have enough money to meet our needs.

But the heart attack shook my confidence about everything. A big part of my fear, fueled by a lack of information, was concern about our financial security. What would happen to our family if my husband were disabled, if he died? Would I have to sell our home? How would I provide the kids with the education we wanted for them? Some days the terror was so bad that I even wondered how we would eat.

One day I stealthily called the Social Security office to find out what benefits our kids would get if he died or were disabled. I was flooded with relief—momentarily. Then I was filled with superstitious fear. Having said the words "disabled" and "die" might magically cause my fears to come true.

You can confront and deal with your fear by strengthening yourself with information, planning for contingencies. Imagining a variety of situations and how you would cope will help you prepare for your changed life, which, hereafter, will include your partner's illness.

Affirmation: I am strong; I will survive and thrive.

Related topics to think/write about:
1) Questions I have about my internal resources and my external circumstances. 2) My feelings about what I don't know enough about, such as finances, work, and so on.

Qualities to meditate on: Confidence–imagination–preparation.

Date _____

This is the ____ _week of my recovery_ _____

_____

_____

_____

_____

_____

_____

_____

_____

_____

_____

_____

_____

_____

_____

_____

_____

_____

_____

_____

_____

_____

_____

_____

_____

_____

_____

_____

_____

_____

_____

_____

_____

_____

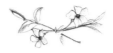

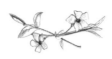

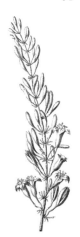

The world breaks everyone, then some become strong at
the broken places.

Ernest Hemingway

Courage is the most obvious quality in the heartmates I have met all around the world. From the very first moment of our partner's diagnosis or health crisis, we summon our courage:

- To face the information about how ill our partner is and what we can expect.
- To visit our mate and maintain our hope.
- To hold our family intact as each member receives the news and joins those waiting in the hospital or at home.
- To acknowledge our feelings—our fear and pain—through our tears and our words.

Facing good or disappointing news requires courage. Peace will elude us if we resist reality.

Affirmation: I have many strengths, including the ability to face reality and uncertainty.

Related topics to think/write about:
1) What is my style of resisting reality? 2) How can I replenish my spirit, which has been severely tested by this crisis?

Qualities to meditate on: Courage–perseverance–realism.

Date _____

This is the _____ *week of my recovery* _____

_____

_____

_____

_____

_____

_____

_____

_____

_____

_____

_____

_____

_____

_____

_____

_____

_____

_____

_____

_____

_____

_____

_____

_____

_____

_____

_____

_____

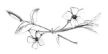

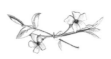

It's important to recognize and be grateful for your partner's
recovery and a return to "normal" living. Celebrate that recovery.
It's also crucial to understand that your transition continues.
What was normal before bears little or no resemblance to life as
you know it today. Some days you will feel great; other days you
won't seem able to pull yourself out of the doldrums.

Rachael Freed
Heartmates

The initial crisis is over and, from the outside, everything seems stable. But on the inside everything feels different. You may wonder, "Why do I feel depressed when my partner's recovering so well? Is there something wrong with me? Now that everyone is so positive and hopeful, why do I feel I can barely make it through the day? Where is my usual energy and enthusiasm for life? Will I ever feel like me again?"

A single word may answer all of these questions: grief. You are in the midst of adapting to change and a new reality, one that includes your partner's illness and all that it implies.

Loss and gain are the two components of change. Losses demand a physical, emotional, mental, and spiritual response. This is grief. There are no shortcuts—we must experience grief to get through it. That's what healing and recovery are all about.

Affirmation: I am capable of experiencing my grief and healing.

Related topics to think/write about:
   1) Things that are different in my life. 2) Nourishing activities for my body, feelings, mind, and soul.

Qualities to meditate on: Strength–surrender–willingness.

Date _____

This is the _____ *week of my recovery* _____

_____

_____

_____

_____

_____

_____

_____

_____

_____

_____

_____

_____

_____

_____

_____

_____

_____

_____

_____

_____

_____

_____

_____

_____

_____

_____

_____

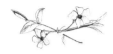

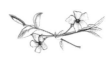

And it is still true, no matter how old you are, when you go out in the world, it is best to hold hands and stick together.
Robert Fulghum

When a health crisis includes hospitalization, you and your mate are separated. From that first night, when you return to a dark house and a cold bed after leaving your partner in the bright, all-night light of the hospital, everything is different. One of you is sick, the other well. Later, when your mate returns home, this separation can include other aspects of your lives: communicating, living a shared vision, intimacy.

The frustration of separation and the yearning to be together is poignant in this example from the television program *thirtysomething:* Nancy has ovarian cancer. Her heartmate, Elliot, tells his friend Al, "It's all about Nancy—you know, 'cuz it has to be. . . . Do you think anyone ever knows how much they're loved? . . . 'Cuz I feel like Nancy's going somewhere and I can't go with her—I can't!" It's true that you can't go on your mate's journey, nor can your mate go on yours. But being partners, talking with each other, can help reduce isolation and deepen the intimacy between you.

It may be difficult to talk about your fear, sadness, and anger. Both of you experienced the shock of the body's betrayal. Both of you face the uncertainty of the future. Suffering the experience in isolation only adds to its difficulty. So hold hands. Talk to each other about your reactions and realizations. You can face your new reality better when you share it. The reward for overcoming isolation is intimacy.

Affirmation: I do not stand alone; I am brave enough to reach out to my partner.

Related topics to think/write about:
1) How have the rules and roles shifted since my mate's illness? 2) How can I balance my need for privacy and my need to feel connected?

Qualities to meditate on: Communication–intimacy–partnership.

*Date*_____

*This is the*_____*week of my recovery*_____

_____

_____

_____

_____

_____

_____

_____

_____

_____

_____

_____

_____

_____

_____

_____

_____

_____

_____

_____

_____

_____

_____

_____

_____

_____

_____

_____

_____

_____

_____

_____

_____

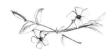

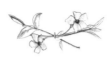

It was very important to explain to my daughter that it wasn't her fault and then let her share in my feelings about being sad, so I didn't have to put on a front that everything was okay when it wasn't.

Robin, a heartmate

It is common for children of all ages to assume that a family tragedy is their fault. "If I hadn't disobeyed him; if I hadn't argued with him the night before . . ." they reason. We need to tell our children clearly and remind them often that what's happened is not their fault.

If you have children, it is impossible to protect them from reality. Masking your anxiety by not talking about Mom's or Dad's illness won't work. Neither will pretending lightness or detachment. Denise Linn, author of *Sacred Legacies,* clarifies that "children know and feel the unspoken; they have an inner radar for the forbidden, dark secrets of a family." Kids easily sense when you're not being straight with them.

They also learn from your behavior and mirror it. If it isn't okay for Mom to express feelings, it must mean that they shouldn't express or even have feelings. If no one lets anyone else know how they feel, there is little opportunity for family members to support each other in this family crisis. Lead by example so your children know that it is normal for everyone in the family to have a whole range of feelings, especially during a crisis.

Affirmation: I protect my children best with my caring and honesty.

Related topics to think/write about:
1) What are my children's needs in this situation? 2) Which needs can I support? 3) Who can meet the needs that I can't?

Qualities to meditate on: Community–harmlessness–integrity.

44

Date _____

This is the _____ *week of my recovery* _____

_____

_____

_____

_____

_____

_____

_____

_____

_____

_____

_____

_____

_____

_____

_____

_____

_____

_____

_____

_____

_____

_____

_____

_____

_____

_____

_____

_____

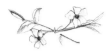

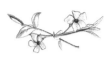

I was dealt a new hand and I didn't know how to play it.
John Updike

One of the hardest things for me about my husband's illness was facing uncertainty. I like to be able to plan; I feel good when I'm in control. In the early days of recovery, I felt insecure and exhausted. And I kept trying to control and manage whatever and whomever I could.

At some point, however, I recalled Mel Brooks' joke about the existence of God in his *2000 and Thirteen-Year-Old Man* album: Phil, worshiped leader of the tribe, was hit by lightning. In awe, one caveman assured another, "There's something bigger than Phil!"

My mate's illness taught me a lesson about my relationship to that "something bigger." Some call it God, others a higher power, the Maker, or life force. Eventually I got the message. I am vulnerable to a future beyond my planning and my personal control. I came to the stark realization that both my husband and I are mortal.

Uncertainty and unpredictability are part of living. They most certainly are part of living with serious illness. Strive for acceptance of this fact of life. Reinhold Niebuhr's Serenity Prayer helps many accept this difficult piece of wisdom:

> God,
> grant me the serenity
> to accept the things I cannot change,
> the courage to change the things I can,
> and the wisdom to know the difference.

Affirmation: I accept the fact of uncertainty, the permanence of change.

Related topics to think/write about:
1) How is it advantageous to know my mate and I are mortal? 2) What are the things I can and can't control?

Qualities to meditate on: Acceptance–serenity–wisdom.

48

Date _____

This is the _____ *week of my recovery* _____

_____

_____

_____

_____

_____

_____

_____

_____

_____

_____

_____

_____

_____

_____

_____

_____

_____

_____

_____

_____

_____

_____

_____

_____

_____

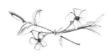

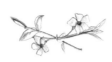

How could this be happening to us? We're too young for this; our family's too young for this. . . . I'm just so angry about how the chips fell the way they did. At the other extreme, I'm so grateful that he is here.

Ethelyn, a heartmate

Our early, natural reactions to a health crisis protect us until the reality can sink in. First there is numbness, shock, denial, and that desperate wish that we will wake up and this nightmare will be over. Some heartmates describe the discomfort as just going through the motions, not really living life. We feel unreal, like our feet aren't connecting us to the earth; our body parts feel unfamiliar or disconnected.

As the days and first weeks pass, the frozen state begins to melt. Shock is replaced by a confusing combination of feelings: anger and gratitude, cheerful optimism and deep disappointment, anxiety and serenity. How is it possible to simultaneously feel so furious and grateful, so relieved and so sad, so fearful and yet peaceful, when the whole situation is beyond our personal control?

The roller coaster of feelings is a normal aspect of the early healing process. As much as you can, recognize the feelings and acknowledge that there is nothing wrong with you. You are not crazy!

Affirmation: My feelings are a normal response to the crisis I am experiencing.

Related topics to think/write about:
Without being concerned with organization, I will write short entries describing my feelings each time I journal this week.

Qualities to meditate on: Comprehension–faith–optimism.

Date _____

This is the _____ *week of my recovery* _____

_____

_____

_____

_____

_____

_____

_____

_____

_____

_____

_____

_____

_____

_____

_____

_____

_____

_____

_____

_____

_____

_____

_____

_____

_____

_____

_____

_____

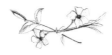

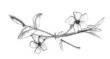

*I went to a lady for a massage one day. I was struck by what a
gentle, loving thing that was. I was so familiar with the feeling of
being deprived of somebody's touch.*

Mary, a heartmate

There is an historic World War II study documenting that babies
in a London orphanage who weren't touched or caressed enough
did not thrive. Although we're not infants, the implications for all
humans, heartmates included, seem clear. In order for us and for
our mates to heal, we need to be touched regularly in positive,
appreciative ways.

The serious illness that separates heartmates and their partners
may erroneously teach us that the patient is too fragile to touch, too
ill to touch us. We may even believe that to arouse our mates sexually
would be dangerous. No wonder we shy away from touching.

It's important to honor this basic human need. Begin to ask for
the touching you need to receive and to give. Revel in touch that
says, "I love you. I'm delighted to be sharing today with you. I'm
glad you are alive!"

Adrienne Rich wrote, "A touch is enough to let us know we're not
alone in the universe, even in sleep." Touching nourishes the spirit and
body of the heartmate. Get a massage. Exchange back rubs with your
mate. Make a daily practice of holding hands and cuddling. Spoon
every night!

Affirmation: I deserve to be touched in loving, respectful ways.

Related topics to think/write about:
1) List obstacles to touching and being touched. 2) What
does it mean to me to be touched lovingly?

Qualities to meditate on: Celebration–generosity–love.

Date _____

This is the _____ week of my recovery _____

_____

_____

_____

_____

_____

_____

_____

_____

_____

_____

_____

_____

_____

_____

_____

_____

_____

_____

_____

_____

_____

_____

_____

_____

_____

_____

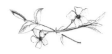

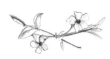

The way we operate is that we use our roles to define ourselves; when parts of our roles are taken away from us, we feel like we're nobody. Men particularly have a problem with that. If masculine functions are taken away they feel diminished.

David Keith, MD
Portrait of the Heartmate

We all feel diminished when our functions at work and at home are usurped as a result of illness. If the patient is accustomed to specific household duties, for example, he or she may be frustrated when the mate assumes these roles. "How can he botch the laundry? Can't she clean right (i.e., my way)?" Lurking under this frustration is the fear of losing one's identity along with one's normal duties.

Heartmates feel frustrated, too. As much as we love our partners, it is difficult to have them around all the time. We go into the kitchen, and there they are—with nothing to do. We need the bathroom to get ready for work, and there they are. It is confusing to feel both grateful for their survival and annoyed at having them underfoot.

Change, whether temporary or permanent, is part of the newness of coping with a severe or chronic illness. It threatens your daily routine, your ability to function, your sense of worth, your very identity. Understanding that all change is stressful may help you to manage better. Take a deep breath; count to ten. Observe what is happening. Acknowledge that change is your reality. Talk about it with your partner. Look for humor in the situation to shift your perspective and aid cooperation.

Affirmation: I am a worthwhile human being who can accommodate change.

Related topics to think/write about:
1) What has changed in my life and how do I feel about those changes? 2) What has changed in my mate's life as a result of the illness?

Qualities to meditate on: Humor–power–resilience.

60

Date _____

This is the _____ *week of my recovery* _____

_____
_____
_____
_____
_____
_____
_____
_____
_____
_____
_____
_____
_____
_____
_____
_____
_____
_____
_____
_____
_____
_____
_____
_____
_____
_____
_____
_____

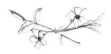

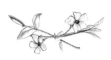

My father seemed so dependent, and I had never ever seen him that way before. It terrified me.

Ellen Sue, daughter of a patient

Children's anxiety about the potential loss of a parent is a powerful catalyst for action. Commonly, kids switch roles and become parents to the parent who is ill. Magical thinking suggests, "If I do for Dad or Mom, nothing bad can happen to them."

This role reversal applies to children both young and old. A year after his mom's stroke, a thirty-year-old son was still visiting every evening after work—completely sacrificing his own social and recreational life. Children reduce their anxiety and express their caring by caretaking. Parents, on the other hand, feel watched, nagged, insulted, and condescended to by overprotective children. In time, children may also feel resentful about their parents' seeming ingratitude and the demands they believe their parents are placing on them.

If you have children, understand that they are adapting to a changed reality based on the serious illness of their parent. Gail A. Noller, PsyD, author of *Finding Your Way: Families and the Cancer Experience,* explains, "When one element [of a family] is suddenly or drastically changed, . . . every element must adapt, must change, in order to find balance again. Restoring balance often takes a long time."

Talk openly with your children about your needs and ask them about theirs. If your children are young, you might seek support for them in the larger community. Ask for and accept help from relatives, friends, coaches, teachers, and clergy. Don't expect yourself to be able to do it all.

Affirmation: I will express my love by stepping back and letting go.

Related topics to think/write about:
1) In what way am I overprotective of my mate and my children? 2) How can I reduce my anxiety without taking responsibility for everything related to my family?

Qualities to meditate on: Cooperation–dedication–responsibility.

64

Date _____

This is the _____ week of my recovery _____

_____

_____

_____

_____

_____

_____

_____

_____

_____

_____

_____

_____

_____

_____

_____

_____

_____

_____

_____

_____

_____

_____

_____

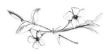

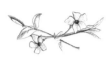

You gain strength, courage, and confidence by every experience in which you really stop to look fear in the face.
Eleanor Roosevelt

Heartmates find themselves faced with two of humanity's deepest fears: fear of being abandoned, and fear for their own survival.

As we confront these fears, we find that we possess great strength and powerful qualities: resilience, perseverance, patience, flexibility, clarity, compassion, and forgiveness. Few of us find ourselves weak; most of us are surprised by our strengths.

Isn't it ironic that we must suffer pain and bear crises to find empowerment and to grow? But it is true: inner strength, like muscular strength, grows when exercised. May we use these newly found and hard-won powers for our own healing and well-being, as well as for our families and others.

Affirmation: I am strong enough to face my fears.

Related topics to think/write about:
1) What are my specific fears? How realistic are they? What can I do so they don't control my life? 2) What are my newfound strengths and how can I use them?

Qualities to meditate on: Liberation–power–understanding.

68

Date _____

This is the _____ *week of my recovery* _____

_____
_____
_____
_____
_____
_____
_____
_____
_____
_____
_____
_____
_____
_____
_____
_____
_____
_____
_____
_____
_____
_____
_____
_____
_____
_____
_____

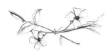

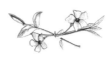

And suddenly you stop and have time to think about the future,
about where your life is going and what changes are going to
happen. For me it was a sudden dip into depression.

                                                    Sharon, a heartmate

Once your early shock and numbness wear off, it is natural and normal to experience exhaustion and depression. Right about this time, your mind may get busy trying to figure out what your new life will be like.

When depression and an innovative mind get together, results can be disastrous. The combination of sadness, disappointment, and catastrophic expectations may suggest to you a bleak future. Strive to remember that these are only fantasies that will probably never come true.

You are aware now, as never before, of how uncertain and fragile life is. Facing so much reality can be frightening, but a crisis also provides opportunity. This can be an important new beginning—a period of reevaluation of your life, your values, and your priorities.

As you turn inward to faith and strength, remember also to reach out to those in your community who can support and encourage your healing.

Affirmation: I am resilient; I can adapt to a life of uncertainty.

Related topics to think/write about:
1) Frightening things my mind says are in my future.
2) What makes me feel sad, disappointed, depressed, powerless?

Qualities to meditate on: Determination–openness–truth.

72

Date _____

This is the _____ *week of my recovery* _____

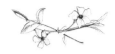

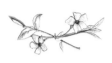

He went through times when he was suffering with depression, having angry feelings, and I guess I thought it was my job to try to control those feelings—to make him happy, cheer him up, try to make him see the positive side of life. I've come to realize that if he wants to feel those feelings, it's all right.

Mary, a heartmate

As a heartmate, much of what you read suggests that optimism and hope will positively affect recovery. Many heartmates believe it is their responsibility to make sure that patients get this message. But the more we teach, preach, cajole, beg, or demand a positive attitude of the patient, the more withdrawn, silent, stubborn, and negative our partner may become.

The fact is that we can't experience or control other people's feelings any more than we can take away their physical pain and spiritual anguish. But we can recognize what we feel when they are angry or depressed. We can talk to ourselves in a positive way. We can take charge of how we respond and react to our feelings. We have choices about how, if, and when we express or don't express our feelings.

As you attend to your feelings, you are taking responsibility for your recovery, furthering your healing. You may find yourself more available and empathetic to your mate, too.

Affirmation: I am responsible for my own feelings, and no one else's.

Related topics to think/write about:
Differentiate my feelings from my mate's by making an annotated list describing how I feel about: my heartmate's illness, the changes in my life, my own grief and recovery.

Qualities to meditate on: Compassion–detachment–harmlessness.

Date _____

This is the ___ *week of my recovery* _____

_____

_____

_____

_____

_____

_____

_____

_____

_____

_____

_____

_____

_____

_____

_____

_____

_____

_____

_____

_____

_____

_____

_____

_____

_____

_____

_____

_____

_____

_____

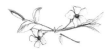

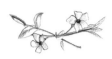

Something that has worked well for many couples is making a pact to share one thing each day that you appreciate about yourselves. That way a realistic and ongoing assessment of your situation can continue. You will also have something worthwhile to talk about every day.

Rachael Freed
Heartmates

An important part of your healing involves "re-pairing" the heartmate connection. Physically separated at the onset of the crisis, each of you had different experiences. With no privacy in the hospital and unsure of your new roles, your communication became stilted. You probably felt like strangers even if you'd been together for fifty years.

Healing is about getting reacquainted, rebuilding the trust in your partnership. Begin to let each other in. Share what happened and what is happening to you, how you feel, what it means. These tiny but significant steps are vital to becoming partners again. Leaving the roles of patient and caretaker, even a few minutes a day, can nourish both of you and give your relationship new life.

Set aside a short time each day just to talk. Plan, share your thoughts, say what you want and need, appreciate yourself and each other. Celebrate your progress together and acknowledge the preciousness of life today.

Affirmation: I will do my part for our partnership.

Related topics to think/write about:
1) Obstacles that make it difficult to trust our partnership.
2) Things I want to share with my mate.

Qualities to meditate on: Friendship–partnership–trust.

Date _____

This is the _____ *week of my recovery* _____

_____

_____

_____

_____

_____

_____

_____

_____

_____

_____

_____

_____

_____

_____

_____

_____

_____

_____

_____

_____

_____

_____

_____

_____

_____

_____

_____

_____

_____

_____

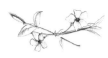

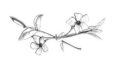

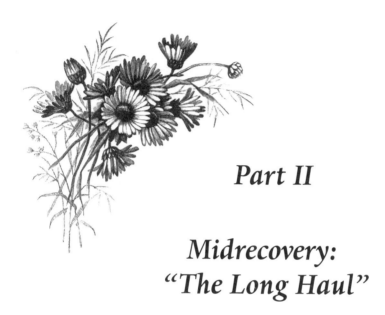

Part II

Midrecovery:
"The Long Haul"

I was definitely the nurse for months after his heart attack, to the point where he would turn to me and say: "Well, do you think I should eat that? Do you think this is too much salt? This would be okay, wouldn't it?" At every turn I was losing my identity as his lover and his wife.

Lavonne, a heartmate

Lavonne's comments speak to issues that occur beyond a heart attack and initial recovery. Things she did for her husband in the acute stage of his illness had become routine and created serious consequences: an imbalance of power and responsibility.

No relationship is perfectly equal, but serious illness does create an imbalance of power and responsibility. The ease with which you integrated caretaking matched your mate's assumption of the role of the patient. This imbalance should not be permanent.

As the patient heals, strive for right responsibility and appropriate roles. Wanting to reclaim your role as partner, for example, is natural and encouraged. To work on reconnecting as mates, explore these activities:

- Talk with your mate about shifting and equalizing responsibility for important lifestyle changes.
- Set aside time to talk about how you can share the responsibilities you took on when your mate became ill.
- Plan time apart so you can each pursue your individual interests.
- Make regular dates to spend time together and share physical affection.

Affirmation: As my mate heals, I will use my power to relinquish control and any temporarily assumed roles.

Related topics to think/write about:
1) In which areas of our lives am I overresponsible or underresponsible? 2) How can we reinvigorate our partner relationship?

Qualities to meditate on: Cooperation–creativity–responsibility.

Date _____

This is the _____ *week of my recovery* _____

_____

_____

_____

_____

_____

_____

_____

_____

_____

_____

_____

_____

_____

_____

_____

_____

_____

_____

_____

_____

_____

_____

_____

_____

_____

_____

_____

_____

_____

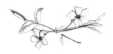

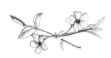

*[Heartmates] share the unique experience of being in a crisis pre-
cipitated by someone else's illness. Your mate is in crisis, too, but
the experience is not the same. You suddenly find yourself in a situation entirely beyond your control that threatens your security
and will change your future.*

Rachael Freed
Heartmates

I've always been most comfortable when I think I'm in control of a situation. As a child I learned to hide my insecure feelings behind a mask of exuberant confidence. I specialized in the things at which I excelled, and I rarely tested myself with goals that went beyond my areas of skill. As an adult, my imperiled feelings buried, I masqueraded as a woman without fear. I shone, sometimes brilliantly, and succeeded at almost everything I did.

My automatic response to my mate's illness was to act as I always had. Only this time it didn't work! His illness was beyond my control and confidence. I drained my energy cheerleading for him, for family, and for friends. All my efforts failed to stop what was happening. I was subject to outside forces that were changing my whole life, and I couldn't predict what was coming.

Perhaps *my* biggest lesson from *his* illness was about learning to accept human limitations—my own and his.

Affirmation: I am human and in the hands of God or my higher power. Or: I am being held by the universe.

Related topics to think/write about:
1) Ways that I can cooperate with what is happening, go with the flow. 2) Recognizing what I can and can't control.

Qualities to meditate on: Letting go–surrender–trust.

Date _____

This is the _____ _week of my recovery_ _____

_____

_____

_____

_____

_____

_____

_____

_____

_____

_____

_____

_____

_____

_____

_____

_____

_____

_____

_____

_____

_____

_____

_____

_____

_____

_____

_____

_____

_____

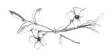

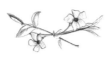

Physicians have always believed in the usefulness and, indeed, the necessity of attitudes as aids in the healing process. . . . Whether this ingredient goes by the name of the patient's own hopefulness or determination or faith or confidence or will to live . . . is not as important as the fact that the positive emotions and attitudes are potent factors in recovery.

Norman Cousins
The Healing Heart

Healing is affected by our optimism and pessimism. Dean Acheson expressed this well: "The manner in which one endures what must be endured is more important than the thing that must be endured."

Learning to think positively increases your control over your perception of your present situation. Your perceptions point to methods you can employ to affect your future. Train yourself to look for and find the positive in your circumstances.

This is not to suggest that you should deny your difficult feelings or the reality of your situation. It simply means that you can choose to focus on the positive or the negative. If you are upset by an event, go a step deeper and consider the cause of the event. You may find that something that seemed a catastrophe is only a minor setback.

Even if your negative belief is accurate, continue to check your attitudes. Ask yourself, "Have I exaggerated the implications? What do the facts really imply? Is my belief destructive to me and my partner? How can I change my belief?" Progress can be measured by how much you focus on solutions and resolutions.

Affirmation: I am learning to think realistically and optimistically.

Related topics to think/write about:
Choose a specific and immediate situation in your life. Analyze your thinking and focus on solutions and resolutions.

Qualities to meditate on: Control–enthusiasm–optimism.

Date _____

This is the _____ *week of my recovery* _____

_____

_____

_____

_____

_____

_____

_____

_____

_____

_____

_____

_____

_____

_____

_____

_____

_____

_____

_____

_____

_____

_____

_____

_____

_____

_____

_____

_____

_____

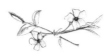

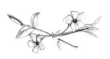

"What am I supposed to do—watch you work yourself to death?
You don't know how much you scare me, Stuart. I lie awake all
night constantly checking to make sure you're still breathing. . . .
I have to keep the TV volume down so I can hear the crash in the
next room when you go down again. I'm scared, Stuart. . . .
I'm just so scared of a life without you."

Anne

LA Law

Sometimes drama is as real as life. In this scene from *LA Law*, heartmate Anne tells her husband, Stuart, about her fear. When the routines we count on for security are shattered by the unexpected, or when we mistake something benign for what we fear most, we respond instantaneously with fear.

The term "vicarious victims of trauma" perfectly fits the heartmate. You are vulnerable as a result of your experience from your partner's health crisis. Your fear doesn't know the difference between burnt toast and the house going up in flames. It is nearly impossible for you to discern a harmless cough from one that sounds like your mate is struggling for his or her last breath.

At times like this, you need to slow down. Take a few deep breaths and ask yourself, "What is really happening here?" Other ways to combat fear include writing about it or talking about it with your mate or a trusted friend.

Affirmation: I can master my fear by recognizing it and assessing real danger.

Related topics to think/write about:
1) Make a list of my questions and where I can get answers. 2) What are my strengths—the ones that have gotten me through other crises in my life?

Qualities to meditate on: Calm–courage–humor.

Date _____

This is the _____ *week of my recovery* _____

_____

_____

_____

_____

_____

_____

_____

_____

_____

_____

_____

_____

_____

_____

_____

_____

_____

_____

_____

_____

_____

_____

_____

_____

_____

_____

_____

_____

_____

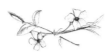

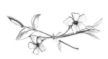

I was being the mother hen . . . and being very intrusive in his life: "Now don't do this, don't do that . . ." and "Do you think you should really do this?" Finally he just told me loud and clear that this wasn't going to be an acceptable lifestyle. I'm slowly finding ways to give up being overprotective and accept his responsibility for his own health and life.

Robin, a heartmate

Many couples are not as open as "mother hen" Robin and her mate, but they often struggle with comparable feelings. If patients are treated like invalids, they will feel invalidated. Stop and think before you rush in to carry something you believe is too heavy or urge your partner to do less because of your fear.

Temporarily taking on more responsibility because of your mate's illness may be necessary. But responsibility laced with fear may quickly become the established way of relating to each other. Temporary emergency measures may crystallize into permanent changes in the division of labor.

With a progressive illness, the changing balance of caregiving makes a respectful relationship between partners difficult to negotiate. For the patient, learning to receive care can be a bumpy road that includes humiliation, shame, guilt, and anger. Identifying, understanding, and negotiating changes in responsibility indicate that you are recovering.

Affirmation: I can differentiate between being rightly responsible and being overresponsible.

Related topics to think/write about:
1) How am I more and less dependent on my mate now?
2) How is my mate more and less dependent on me?
3) How do I feel about my responsibilities since the onset of my partner's illness?

Qualities to meditate on: Freedom–goodwill–responsibility.

*Date*_____

*This is the*_____ *week of my recovery*_____

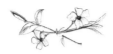

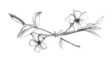

We've found that the longer we're together and the closer we are, the more ways there are to make love and to love each other without actually having intercourse. Both of us feel satisfied and very, very close.

Dorothy, a heartmate

Many patients *are* physically capable of returning to their normal sexual practices after surgery, during rehabilitation, or in periods of remission. But sexual dysfunction, whether caused by medications, depression, or fear, is a real problem for many couples. Sexual dysfunction can activate a heartmate's fear of rejection, of feeling unloved, of deprivation. At the same time, you may fear that the stress of having intercourse is too dangerous to risk. Moreover, it's hard to make love when you have not voiced your feelings of fear, anger, and resentment.

Your sexual needs may be in flux along with your values and priorities. This may be the single most difficult subject to talk about with healthcare professionals, friends, even with your partner. If a long-term physical result of the illness is lost or reduced sexuality, you need to mourn that loss. But rarely is it necessary to abandon sexual intimacy altogether.

Communication is the key to returning to loving physical intimacy. Acknowledge your need for physical closeness. Ask for what you want. Experiment: find satisfying ways to be intimate that fit your specific circumstances.

Affirmation: I am loving, lovable, and desirable.

Related topics to think/write about:
1) Things I want to discuss with my partner. 2) Ways we can celebrate our partnership.

Qualities to meditate on: Friendship–love–tenderness–trust.

Date _____

This is the _____ *week of my recovery* _____

_____

_____

_____

_____

_____

_____

_____

_____

_____

_____

_____

_____

_____

_____

_____

_____

_____

_____

_____

_____

_____

_____

_____

_____

_____

_____

_____

_____

_____

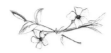

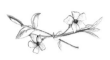

Partners need to find ways to care for themselves. Being a full-time caregiver is exhausting and wears thin. . . . Take breaks from the role. . . . Don't feel guilty about enjoying work . . . away from the pressure and the strain of home. . . . Feel[ing] re-involved with life again . . . represents the choice you have made to become better rather than bitter.

> Gail A. Noller, PsyD
> *Finding Your Way:*
> *Families and the Cancer Experience*

It seems overwhelming to wean yourself from the all-encompassing role of caregiver and to reinvest in your own life. It's frightening to be gone for an hour to buy groceries, let alone to leave your recovering partner for a day or overnight.

Activities that were a normal part of your life before the illness may now seem unimportant or frivolous. Social engagements may take too much energy, energy you just don't have. A fascinating book requires too much effort, and you have neither the concentration nor the interest.

At every turn, you are fearful. The familiar is no longer comforting; the new has its own hazards. You wonder what is wrong—whether you've gone crazy. Will life ever seem predictable again?

You have not gone crazy! It takes many weeks and months to grieve your losses and establish a new normal, one that includes the illness as well as other important aspects of your life. Take your time; don't be pressured by others. Grief is unique to each of us. Let your interest and energy level guide your return to functioning in the larger world.

Affirmation: I trust my own pace.

Related topics to think/write about:
    1) List things that are important and unimportant now. I may want to do this every month for some time to recognize my progress. 2) Make a graduated plan and timetable for returning to outside activities.

Qualities to meditate on: Balance–energy–realism.

110

Date _____

This is the ____ *week of my recovery* _____

_____

_____

_____

_____

_____

_____

_____

_____

_____

_____

_____

_____

_____

_____

_____

_____

_____

_____

_____

_____

_____

_____

_____

_____

_____

_____

_____

_____

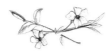

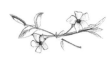

Illness, and perhaps only illness, gives us permission to slow down. . . . Illness restores the sense of proportion that is lost when we take life for granted.

Arthur W. Frank, a cancer
and heart patient
At the Will of the Body

Must we be in crisis to hear the wisdom in the old adage, "Take time to smell the roses"? Why not walk in the sunlight, hear the birds, appreciate sunrise and sunset? Nature is free and available to us in all its abundance. To be nourished by nature, all we need to do is awaken to it. Rushing through each day, trying to "do it all," we miss what's essential: Being here. Now.

When the present is difficult or we are afraid of what's happening, we often try to fix it or avoid it. We focus on the past, yearning for what's lost, or concentrate on the future, wishing for something to look forward to—anything but what's happening now.

Michael Landon told it straight: "Somebody should tell us, right at the start of our lives, that we are dying. Then we might live life to the limit, every minute of every day." Staying in the moment is how we live life fully, even when that moment of our life is difficult.

Coming to terms with your new reality will be easier if you look for the positive, the precious, and feel grateful for what you have today. In order to have "now," you need only remember a few simple things:

- Now is all we really have.
- Focus on who and what is available to you now.
- Fill yourself full with the abundance of the moment.
- Experience gratitude for being alive right now.

Affirmation: I rejoice in the blessings of my life today.

Related topics to think/write about:
1) What do I find positive and precious in my life? 2) Who and what nurtures me?

Qualities to meditate on: Acceptance–appreciation–gratitude.

*Date*_____

This is the _____ *week of my recovery*_____

_____

_____

_____

_____

_____

_____

_____

_____

_____

_____

_____

_____

_____

_____

_____

_____

_____

_____

_____

_____

_____

_____

_____

_____

_____

_____

_____

_____

_____

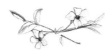

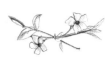

*You can change the way you cook, and you can adjust to coming
home earlier on Saturday night. . . . You can learn to live with less
money, and you will still be you. But the changes that [heartmates]
experience go deeper. They affect the very center of your identity.*

Rachael Freed
Heartmates

People commonly identify themselves according to their responsibilities, the roles they play in daily life—what they do, not who they are. But a health crisis is an uncommon experience and a powerful invitation to discover a deeper identity.

We tell and retell the story of what's happened, we recall earlier losses, all in an attempt to understand the meaning of this event in our lives. We clarify our values; we hone and refine our priorities.

We peel away our outer layers in search of our core. We find the reality of our own mortality as well as our partner's. In understanding limitation, some of us find or deepen our faith in the immortality of our souls. Others find a spiritual connection in surrendering to the mystery of life and death.

Your partner's illness is a catalyst for spiritual development. Personal and spiritual growth are the greatest opportunities available to us as we grieve the losses inherent in a health crisis.

Affirmation: I am more than what I do.

Related topics to think/write about:
1) Write "my" story of my partner's illness, focusing on the changes I recognize in my own life. 2) List changes in my values and priorities since my mate became ill.

Qualities to meditate on: Comprehension–faith–wonder.

Date _____

This is the _____ *week of my recovery* _____

_____

_____

_____

_____

_____

_____

_____

_____

_____

_____

_____

_____

_____

_____

_____

_____

_____

_____

_____

_____

_____

_____

_____

_____

_____

_____

_____

_____

_____

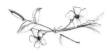

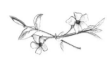

I went with my daughters to the park. I watched them playing; they were so small and at such a neat age. I remember seeing people riding by on bicycles, whole families—husbands, wives, small children. And suddenly it hit me—we may never get to do that again!

Lavonne, a heartmate

Months have passed since your mate became ill, and your new lifestyle is becoming routine. Yet your recovery is slowed because you're still mourning the loss of your "normal" life, life as it was before the disease. Everyday events unexpectedly trigger your mourning: a physical activity like family biking, the weekend ritual of your grandkids playing horsy with your mate.

So many heartmates use their energy trying to recreate life as it was before the onset of the illness. But it's not possible: everything is different. Let yourself feel your losses. Until you do, you won't be able to construct "the new normal." Your family's new normal is different from that of other families' because you and your situation are unique. Yet, you are not alone. There are similarities in the challenge that all families experience as they adapt to a new normal that includes serious illness.

Be gentle with yourself as you adapt to the changes. Allow yourself to feel, and make space and time for the real sadness in your life. Shed tears if they're there, write about it, tell a friend, and know that, as with all feelings, your sadness, too, shall pass.

Affirmation: I am strong enough to experience my sadness and my disappointment.

Related topics to think/write about:
1) The positive and negative aspects of the changes I am making in my life. 2) My feelings about family changes brought on by the illness and its consequences.

Qualities to meditate on: Creativity–determination–flexibility.

122

Date _____

This is the _____ _week of my recovery_ _____

_____

_____

_____

_____

_____

_____

_____

_____

_____

_____

_____

_____

_____

_____

_____

_____

_____

_____

_____

_____

_____

_____

_____

_____

_____

_____

_____

_____

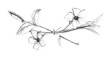

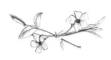

Sometimes the loneliness comes from not having anyone to share
pleasure with: a woman . . . says that when they went on vaca-
tion, "I went with M. and he went with his multiple sclerosis."
                                              Maggie Strong
                                              Mainstay

Whether it is the adventure of a new place, the joy of a warm get-away during the cold winter, the relaxation of a weekend spent fishing and walking in the woods, or the love of a visit with the grandchildren, yours is a lonely dream. Sometimes our partners just won't go. If they do, they seem to have lost their ability to have fun, relax, or be playful.

Safety may be their first priority. They may be afraid to be farther than a phone call away from the doctor and hospital. Or they may see spending money on "pleasure" as wasteful.

In your loneliness it may feel like you're struggling against an invisible but powerful seduction, one that has taken your mate's attention, your closeness, even your physical intimacy. Your mate is engaged, but not with you. It feels like you've lost your partnership.

You can talk directly with your mate, bringing the fears lurking in the shadows out into the light. Your partner's recovery is important, but it also is important to tell him or her that you have needs, too.

You can begin to go places and do things alone. Being by yourself is not necessarily lonely, although it's different than the experience of doing things with your partner. You can make plans with friends and find pleasure beyond your heartmate relationship. You can continue to suggest things you can do as a couple that meet both your needs.

Affirmation: I am entitled to experience the abundance of life.

Related topics to think/write about:
1) What is the difference between being alone and being lonely?
2) How comfortable am I with being alone? 3) How do I handle loneliness in my life?

Qualities to meditate on: Abundance–adventure–play.

Date _____

This is the _____ _week of my recovery_ _____

_____

_____

_____

_____

_____

_____

_____

_____

_____

_____

_____

_____

_____

_____

_____

_____

_____

_____

_____

_____

_____

_____

_____

_____

_____

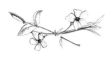

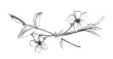

Now I don't feel anxious that if I'm not there and awake every minute, he'll die. I used to feel I couldn't leave to do anything, because then if something happened, I wouldn't be there to take care of it. Now I know I can't keep the inevitable from happening to anybody; none of us can.

Dorothy, a heartmate

The overresponsibility this heartmate conquered is familiar to all of us. Earlier she was angry, frightened, discouraged, and exhausted. Her serenity makes us wonder, How did she make the shift, let go, surrender? How long will it take me to have the wisdom she possesses?

I'm reminded of another heartmate who complained about having to change her cooking style: "I really resented having to cook without salt, not eat beef . . . but eventually, when you stop fighting things, it gets a lot easier." That's the key to surrendering, to letting go: stop fighting reality. But how?

Recognizing and expressing feelings, verbally or on paper, always precedes acceptance and integration. Over time, both of these heartmates expressed their feelings of fear and rage, sadness and disappointment. Liberated from the stranglehold of those feelings, both heartmates arrived at a new perspective, an appreciation for the preciousness of what they had, individually and with their partners.

Affirmation: I will respectfully acknowledge my feelings without judgment.

Related topics to think/write about:
1) My strong feelings, particularly those I disapprove of.
2) Safe and harmless ways to express my feelings.

Qualities to meditate on: Acceptance–detachment–serenity–understanding.

130

Date _____

This is the ____ week of my recovery _____

_____
_____
_____
_____
_____
_____
_____
_____
_____
_____
_____
_____
_____
_____
_____
_____
_____
_____
_____
_____
_____
_____
_____
_____
_____
_____
_____
_____
_____
_____

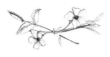

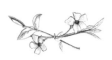

Mourning makes peace with change.
Grief does not have to do with despair.
Yakima Indian Nation

In *Fear of Fifty*, Erica Jong argues the right of her friend to grieve: "Everyone wanted her to perk up. . . . But she needed to mourn. Her need was made more painful by the denial of death that pervades our culture. 'Dust yourself off and go on,' said the collective voice of collective wisdom. 'Haven't you been grieving an awfully long time. . . ?' How they dared to judge another's grief I did not know." Heartmates everywhere deserve such a forceful supporter and advocate.

Grief will not succumb to the pressure of our society. It will not be reduced by force. It will not be hurried. It will not yield its lessons or its gifts instantaneously.

Grief takes time, reflection, and experience. Tell your story again and again. Shed tears for your losses. Update your images and accept human limitations, your own and your mate's. Your body, feelings, mind, and spirit can accommodate the monumental lessons offered by the crisis as you discover and accept what is new—but only over time.

Each person's pace and style of grieving is unique. Take the time you need to grieve in the ways that feel right to you, trusting that your grief will ease and that you will be made better for it. Good grief!

Affirmation: I will honor my grief by giving myself the time I need.

Related topics to think/write about:
1) My image of who I was, and who my mate was, before the onset of this illness. 2) The losses I have mourned, am mourning, and have left to mourn.

Qualities to meditate on: Identity–integrity–meaning.

134

Date _____

This is the _____ *week of my recovery* _____

_____
_____
_____
_____
_____
_____
_____
_____
_____
_____
_____
_____
_____
_____
_____
_____
_____
_____
_____
_____
_____
_____
_____
_____
_____
_____
_____
_____
_____

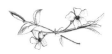

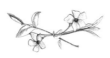

I emphasize finding sources of pleasure. I've had people reject that idea, saying, "Are you telling me to have fun at this terrible moment?" But that moment is life. . . . The more you can become "unfused," lovingly detached, and the more outlets and pleasure you can find, the more you have energy and love and emotions to give to the person who is disabled.

Clara Livsey, MD
from *Mainstay*

Rejecting pleasure can be a way to avoid feeling guilty. It can be a way of dealing with your fear that if you feel happy, people will cease to support you and may even condemn you. It's common to think: "How can I consider my own pleasure when my mate is ill? Only bad and selfish people would enjoy themselves in such a circumstance."

But let's look at the matter logically. Does denying yourself pleasure help your mate? Your partner may survive for another thirty years or more. Is it appropriate to avoid pleasure just to protect your image of selflessness?

If you choose to stay wholeheartedly in the relationship when your mate becomes ill, it becomes even more important for you to develop your individuality, your wholeness. If you don't, you will become invisible and actually experience yourself disappearing in his or her illness.

Starving your heart and soul, denying yourself the beauty and pleasures of life, will only make you unhealthy, resentful, and bitter. Nourishing your heart and soul will lead you to share joy and love with your partner, energizing your relationship.

Affirmation: I will enjoy this moment.

Related topics to think/write about:
1) The activities and things that give me pleasure. 2) Plans for including small, realistic pleasures in my day.

Qualities to meditate on: Beauty–joy–light–play.

138

Date _____

This is the _____ *week of my recovery* _____

_____

_____

_____

_____

_____

_____

_____

_____

_____

_____

_____

_____

_____

_____

_____

_____

_____

_____

_____

_____

_____

_____

_____

_____

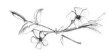

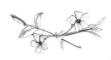

He still feels more comfortable asking me whether or not it's safe
for him to eat something. I have difficulty knowing how I can get
away from that responsibility. I was perhaps too eager to take on
the job at the beginning and now I would like to unload it.

Gretchen, a heartmate

Enabling your partner to remain helpless isn't healthy for either of you or for your relationship. The role of "patient" is emotionally destructive over the long haul, and may even slow your mate's physical recovery. Some people feel safer, more "loved" if they're babied, but they also resent their loss of power and responsibility. Even when your efforts are motivated by caring and concern, taking on too much responsibility may backfire, trapping you into doing more than you should.

If you try to carry children once they've learned to walk on their own, they often respond by kicking you. The same letting go you may have learned as a parent applies to reestablishing a partner relationship with your recovering mate.

A combination of rest and responsibility is the best way for your mate to regain strength and confidence. And your recovery depends on reestablishing a balance of power and responsibility in relation to your strengths and limitations.

Affirmation: My mate and I are separate, each of us individual and whole.

Related topics to think/write about:
1) My style of encouraging helplessness and ways I can let go of it. 2) My ideal of sharing responsibility and power in my heartmate relationship.

Qualities to meditate on: Empowerment–responsibility–surrender.

142

Date _____

This is the _____ *week of my recovery* _____

_____
_____
_____
_____
_____
_____
_____
_____
_____
_____
_____
_____
_____
_____
_____
_____
_____
_____
_____
_____
_____
_____
_____
_____
_____
_____
_____
_____
_____
_____

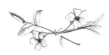

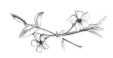

Disease is a simple fact of life, and the older we get, the more
likely we are to become ill with something or other. Our challenge
now, as conscious beings, is how to meet these changes wisely. We
need to plan for how we'll deal with a serious illness, because
sooner or later it will happen to most of us.

> Ram Dass, a stroke patient
> *Still Here*

My friend Shussie, whose husband, Al, recently suffered a painfully debilitating attack of shingles, said, "I'm trying to be as empathic as I can—it could have gone the other way. I would hope if and when it does, he'll be there for me." You may not be able to plan whether you will be the heartmate or the patient, but understanding, compassion, and love will go a long way when you or your partner become ill.

You can't change what has already happened to you and your mate. You can't even change how you feel about it. But you can choose the attitude you will take toward what is happening, the way you accept this new reality, and how you treat yourself and your mate. In *We Are Not Alone: Learning to Live with Chronic Illness,* Sefra Kobrin Pitzele advises: "Be patient with each other. . . . Begin by expecting the best and preparing for the worst. Give courage to each other. There will be good times, too. When all the chores are done and you are both well-rested, remember to do something nice for each other. Keep working to make your relationship better."

Affirmation: I will pay attention to what my mate's illness has to teach me.

Related topics to think/write about:
1) How to deal emotionally and spiritually with my partner and his or her illness. 2) My ideas about the nature of illness and spiritual healing. What do I need now for my own healing?

Qualities to meditate on: Compassion–meaning–partnership.

Date _____

This is the _____ *week of my recovery* _____

_____

_____

_____

_____

_____

_____

_____

_____

_____

_____

_____

_____

_____

_____

_____

_____

_____

_____

_____

_____

_____

_____

_____

_____

_____

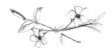

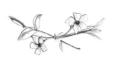

For there is nothing to guarantee that we will be able to remain long enough or deeply enough in front of the unknown, a psychological state that the traditional paths have always recognized as sacred. In that fleeting state . . . [a person] is said to be able to receive the truth, both about nature and his own possible role in the universal order.

Jacob Needleman
A Sense of the Cosmos

Heartmates live in the face of the unknown. We don't know if or how our partner will recover, nor do we know how we will respond to the demands of the illness minute to minute. Living with uncertainty is by far the most difficult challenge of any serious illness, and doing so often requires faith and courage beyond what we believe we possess.

You have had no choice about being "in front of the unknown" in relation to your mate's illness. But there is a lesson you can take from your experience: you have not only survived the challenge, but come through the crisis strengthened.

Your newfound courage gives you the ability and skills to confront the unknown in a broader context. It is the stepping stone to the sacred, the mystery of life.

Affirmation: I commit myself to the spiritual task of opening to the unknown.

Related topics to think/write about:
1) My thoughts, images, and feelings about not knowing, about uncertainty. 2) My thoughts about the universal order and my role in it.

Qualities to meditate on: Order–strength–universality.

*Date*_____

This is the _____ *week of my recovery* _____

_____
_____
_____
_____
_____
_____
_____
_____
_____
_____
_____
_____
_____
_____
_____
_____
_____
_____
_____
_____
_____
_____
_____
_____
_____

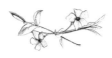

152

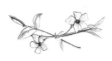

I am dying inside if I don't take care of myself. . . . How can I hold on to myself and love her?

Greg, a heartmate

One of the most painful tasks of the well partner is to accept that you *are* well and live in the well world. This must be balanced with the reality that you love and live with someone whose world is, to some extent, the world of illness.

You do not make your partner well if you deny your wellness or ignore your own needs. Nor can you bypass your guilt about being well (similar to the guilt expressed by survivors of accidents, fires, attacks, or wars) by avoiding reality, pretending the difference doesn't exist.

Your mate's illness may set you both up to believe that he or she has all the weaknesses and you have all the strengths. You want to utilize your competence on your partner's behalf, but you also need the freedom to share your limitations: your shrinking patience, your irritation and resentment, your disappointment. Expressing your weaknesses testifies to your humanity and may give your partner permission to accept his or her own humanity, strengths, and weaknesses.

Taking care of yourself, which is defined differently by every heartmate, is not selfish. It is an absolute necessity in order for you to thrive. Without that foundation, you will not be able to love or care for your mate.

Affirmation: I will love myself and my mate.

Related topics to think/write about:
1) What are my strengths? What do I need as I face the reality of my mate's illness? 2) What do I need to find mental, emotional, and spiritual balance? 3) What do I need to find balance in my relationship with my partner?

Qualities to meditate on: Generosity–harmony–peace.

Date _____

This is the _____ _week of my recovery_ _____

_____

_____

_____

_____

_____

_____

_____

_____

_____

_____

_____

_____

_____

_____

_____

_____

_____

_____

_____

_____

_____

_____

_____

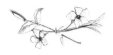

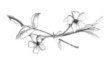

I found myself looking at my life, saying, "I may be sole support here before long." I didn't trust him. I didn't trust his health anymore.
                                                    Mary, a heartmate

Before they became ill, we might have described our partners as stalwart, rugged, or vigorous, even though somewhere deep inside we knew they were also human and mortal. It is common to acknowledge strong images and ignore the fragility of life.

But the shock of a serious diagnosis shatters the trust we've built over many years. We feel betrayed. Once we know that our partner's body, health, and life are vulnerable, our image of his or her invincibility is lost. We may even vow not to feel close to our mate again to avoid the pain of a future betrayal.

Can we regain trust? Trust, based on experience, can only be rebuilt one step at a time and in keeping with the reality of the present moment. Define carefully what you can trust each day. For example, as your mate continues to recover or completes treatment, you can trust that he or she will awaken each morning, that his or her endurance and strength are returning, and so on.

Life is ephemeral. To prepare yourself for a variety of possibilities, ask all the questions you have. Seek all the information you need. Plan for a variety of contingencies. Talk about your experience of trust, both its loss and rediscovery, with your mate and with an understanding friend.

Affirmation: I will open myself to realistic trust.

Related topics to think/write about:
1) Things I trust about myself and my mate. 2) My feelings about betrayal and my fear of being abandoned.

Qualities to meditate on: Clarity–faith–love–trust.

158

Date _____

This is the _____ *week of my recovery* _____

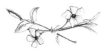

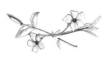

I'm angry at his bad genes, and I'm angry that he doesn't watch his diet like he should. I have trouble separating out what is his right to do as an adult, what is his obligation to me, being married, and what he owes me as a spouse.

Yleen, a heartmate

Anger is a much-criticized emotion, especially in women. Women are told it's not ladylike, it's unattractive, it turns others off or pushes them away.

Anger is a normal part of grief following a health crisis. For heartmates who often feel depressed, lethargic, or hopeless, anger can be a blessing. Anger is a hot energy that fires the power to act.

Anger is usually my first response when something unjust happens. It leads me to react to the injustice rather than feel hopeless in the face of it. Other times my anger is like the surface of a wound, visible and ugly. It covers a hurt or sadness that I find difficult to accept, and at those times anger is my defense.

You have no option about whether you *feel* angry or not. But you do have a choice about whether to utilize the energy of your anger in a positive, constructive way. Doing so is within your capabilities.

Be as respectful as you can of your anger and the anger of others, even if it doesn't feel good or make logical sense to you. Remember that anger is only a feeling, but a feeling that is telling you something. Use your anger in healthy, beneficial ways. Channel its energy to help you, your partner, and your family to heal.

Affirmation: I will use the energy of my anger constructively.

Related topics to think/write about:
1) Examine my past and present attitudes about my anger. 2) New ideas for utilizing the energy of my anger.

Qualities to meditate on: Discernment–energy–vitality.

162

Date _____

This is the ___ *week of my recovery* _____

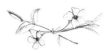

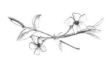

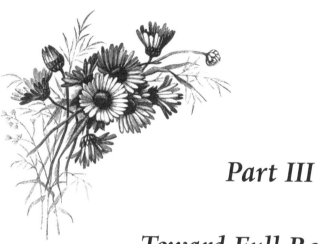

Part III

Toward Full Recovery:
"I Can See the Light"

We find that the lesson we learn again and again is that of accepting heroic helplessness.

Florida Scott-Maxwell
The Measure of My Days

Our family's health crisis, prompted by the onset of my husband's illness, turned out to be a gift for me. I certainly didn't experience it as a gift during the early months when I was terrified and striving to hold everything together all by myself, nor while I was filled with a sense of responsibility for children and a sick husband. In those days I was blinded by outdated visions of heroism, old standards of action and control, and the illusion of power.

Becoming a heartmate, I learned to recognize and accept my helplessness. It was a turning point in my life; I became a different kind of heroine. I developed the courage to face what can only be faced alone: the meaning and purpose of *my* life, the significance of *my* life, and *my* own mortality.

Paradoxically, as I confronted those questions alone, a whole community opened to me. I found cooperation and connection more attractive than the external world of competition and competence. More whole within myself, I sought to deepen my relationships with others and with the God of my understanding.

Affirmation: I am whole and a part of creation.

Related topics to think/write about:
1) The lessons that my partner's illness has taught me thus far. 2) How my values and priorities have changed since my mate became ill.

Qualities to meditate on: Cooperation–harmony–wholeness.

168

Date _____

This is the _____ *week of my recovery* _____

_____

_____

_____

_____

_____

_____

_____

_____

_____

_____

_____

_____

_____

_____

_____

_____

_____

_____

_____

_____

_____

_____

_____

_____

_____

_____

_____

_____

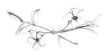

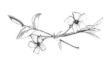

When I think about my friends, they think about their parents as permanent people—I think about my parents as temporary!
Sid, son of a patient

When there is a life-threatening illness in the family, children of every age confront the reality that their parents are mortal. Early images of parents usually include superhuman qualities. Serious or chronic illness requires kids to rework their images to better match reality.

Children, like adults, respond to crisis uniquely. Some are eager to talk about it; some never do. Many will alter their life choices: going away to school or not, marrying or remaining single, taking over the parent's business, moving to a different part of the country, having their own children early or late, and so on.

As you learn the lesson of mortality, you help your children indirectly. You affect the family climate in the way you respond to the new reality of a serious illness. It's good to remember that an illness is one important aspect of the family, but it isn't the family's sole concern.

Another bittersweet but important lesson is that it's impossible to protect children from reality. Perhaps it was my own denial of death that made me say, "They were too young to have to learn that." Years later, I see that the lessons our children learned were crucial in defining who they have become. They are careful about maintaining healthy lifestyles; their priorities and choices are measured in part by their first-hand experience with illness and the reality of mortality. Most important, their awareness of and gratitude for the blessings of their lives and appreciation for their parents color their faith and their actions.

Affirmation: I celebrate the love and learning given me in my life as a parent.

Related topics to think/write about:
1) The most important lessons about parenting that I learned from my mate's illness. 2) Things I want to discuss with my children.

Qualities to meditate on: Faith–gratitude–responsibility.

Date _____

This is the   _week of my recovery_ _____

_____

_____

_____

_____

_____

_____

_____

_____

_____

_____

_____

_____

_____

_____

_____

_____

_____

_____

_____

_____

_____

_____

_____

_____

_____

_____

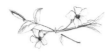

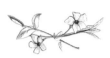

Courage is resistance to fear, mastery of fear—not absence of fear.
Mark Twain

The question I'm asked most often in my work with heartmates is, "When will the fear go away?" Here's my answer: You have been wounded by your mate's health crisis. Wounds scar over with time. You will have your scars and the wounds buried beneath them for the rest of your days. Over time, the scars will fade and your fears will diminish. But if your routine is shattered again by something unexpected, the wounds will burst open and you will suffer fear as if it were the original event all over again.

Away from home at a professional conference, I returned to my hotel room between meetings late one morning. The phone's message light was pulsing. I was instantly paralyzed with fear. Who would call long distance in the morning? Only someone with terrible news!

I reached for the phone, and it seemed an eternity until the operator returned with my message. It was from my kids, and it began with the words, "Sorry if we scared you, but there is good news. . . ." I was limp and exhausted when I hung up the phone. My body and feelings responded to the unexpected as if it were a medical emergency, not a happy message.

Affirmation: I am strong enough to feel and master my fears.

Related topics to think/write about:
1) Describe in detail my five greatest fears. 2) Ways I have dealt with and can deal with the unexpected.

Qualities to meditate on: Courage–realism–serenity.

Date _____

This is the ___ *week of my recovery* _____

_____

_____

_____

_____

_____

_____

_____

_____

_____

_____

_____

_____

_____

_____

_____

_____

_____

_____

_____

_____

_____

_____

_____

_____

_____

_____

_____

_____

_____

_____

_____

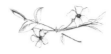

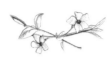

One day I left the hospital with the feeling of: "Okay, this is our life and doggone we're really going to enjoy it. I'm going to quit running around frantically finding a new doctor, a new drug, a new fixit. I'm just going to relax and enjoy what we have." And it was just like a weight had left me after all those years.

Dorothy, a heartmate

Major tasks of grieving include acknowledging your feelings and figuring out how to make lifestyle changes. The work is exhausting. You're engaged in a powerful and lonely struggle. You may be the sole caregiver advocating for your mate in the health system, as well as the family breadwinner, a parent or grandparent, and the child of an aging parent. It's especially difficult to have so much responsibility when you feel isolated and misunderstood, fatigued and unappreciated. Unlike a bad dream that disappears in the light, the reality of your mate's illness is still there when you wake up each day.

In many cases, it is absolutely right that you take the responsibility of being your mate's defender. Some patients are too ill or weak to be their own advocate. There comes a time, however, after many months and sometimes years, when you stop struggling and experience acceptance. Your partner's recovery or quality of life may not be what you had hoped. Acceptance involves knowing that you can't be responsible for another person's life, and that you can't protect your mate from death.

With acceptance comes peace—and forgiveness for your mate and yourself. Surprisingly, you now have renewed energy for life and a new perspective. You begin to embrace gratitude for the precious moments and days you still have to share.

Affirmation: I accept my strengths and my limitations.

Related topics to think/write about:
1) Things I've been frantic about that I can consider letting go. 2) My sense of gratitude, forgiveness, even joy.

Qualities to meditate on: Acceptance–forgiveness–peace.

Date _____

This is the _____ *week of my recovery* _____

_____

_____

_____

_____

_____

_____

_____

_____

_____

_____

_____

_____

_____

_____

_____

_____

_____

_____

_____

_____

_____

_____

_____

_____

_____

_____

_____

_____

_____

_____

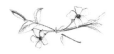

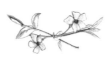

The stereotype of the "good woman" . . . is a portrait of a gentle, sweet, even-tempered, and, inherently, long-suffering woman. Many women have been conditioned to strive for this ideal, and they struggle to maintain such a picture of themselves, even during a crisis. . . . [The "good woman"] doesn't know she has needs. She doesn't know that recovery from her crisis demands that she take care of herself.

Rachael Freed
Heartmates

You may have grown up in an age when women's worth was measured by how well they cared for their men and their children. But times have changed, and we have come of age. Today, women and men have broader opportunities to develop as full human beings. Our lives have purpose and meaning beyond the caregiver role.

We may have given more than half our lives to caring for others. But at middle age we are pregnant with ourselves, creative in ways we never dreamed of in youth. We have both roots and wings.

Being in a relationship always makes the achievement of individual goals more complicated, but it does not invalidate our need for our own lives. We must not let our mate's illness become a barrier that excludes us from the challenge of being and becoming ourselves.

Affirmation: I redefine myself as I integrate my worthiness.

Related topics to think/write about:
1) What are my individual opportunities at my age and in my situation? 2) How do I want to express who I am?

Qualities to meditate on: Authenticity–creativity–integrity.

Date _____

This is the _____ *week of my recovery* _____

_____

_____

_____

_____

_____

_____

_____

_____

_____

_____

_____

_____

_____

_____

_____

_____

_____

_____

_____

_____

_____

_____

_____

_____

_____

_____

_____

_____

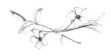

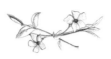

One of the things that happened in our family is that suddenly we were all aware of our mortality. Our children were aware—maybe not so much of their mortality, but of ours. And even though it's such a painful thing, there's a special bond in the family. It's a deep appreciation of each other.

Mary, a heartmate

I have heard heartmates describe their partner's life-threatening illness as the best thing that ever happened—a kind of wake-up call. The awakening was about love and the meaning of relationships, about mortality and the preciousness of life, about making time and space in life to experience the new, the important, the intimate.

But first you must grieve the loss of the old life and the old dreams. Generally this takes at least a year, so that all family occasions, seasons, and holidays will become part of the new reality. As this process nears completion, your attention begins to shift from grieving what was lost to realizing the new opportunities presented to you.

Your energy level informs you when you've grieved enough. You awaken with an interest in the day ahead of you. Your humor and sense of perspective return. You once again think about and plan for your future.

Affirmation: I am preparing myself to live fully in the present by grieving past losses.

Related topics to think/write about:
1) My thoughts about the gift of life. 2) How I want to live from this day forward.

Qualities to meditate on: Appreciation–humor–playfulness.

188

Date _____

This is the _____ _week of my recovery_ _____

_____

_____

_____

_____

_____

_____

_____

_____

_____

_____

_____

_____

_____

_____

_____

_____

_____

_____

_____

_____

_____

_____

_____

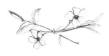

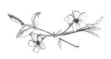

Teach us to face life with faith and courage that we may see the blessings hidden away, even in its discords and struggles. Life calls us not merely to enjoy the beauties that surround us, but to exult in heights attained after the toil of climbing. Grief is a great teacher, when it sends us back to serve and bless the living.
Rabbi Max A. Shapiro

Years ago my rabbi told me he had counseled many bereaved people in his job as a clergyman, but not until his own beloved wife died did he really understand the losses of his congregation. As a clinical social worker, I, too, have guided people in relation to various losses, but being a heartmate taught me a depth of compassion and understanding I could only have learned through experience. Thank you, God, for blessing me with gifts that enable me to help others heal.

Grieving the losses inherent in your crisis has changed you. You can be more compassionate toward yourself about your own limitations and failings. You can be more tolerant about your mate's struggles as well. You can be more understanding as you support your children. As you touch others in your community, they, too, will benefit from your experience with grief.

As Elisabeth Kübler-Ross, our culture's pioneer in understanding grief, wrote, "The ultimate lesson all of us have to learn is unconditional love, which includes not only others but ourselves."

Affirmation: I will live as a blessing to myself and those around me.

Related topics to think/write about:
1) The blessings I found in struggling with my mate's illness.
2) What grief has taught me.

Qualities to meditate on: Compassion–education–service.

192

Date _____

This is the _____ *week of my recovery* _____

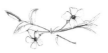

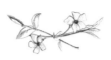

Many times a day I realize how much my outer and inner life is built upon the labors of others, both living and dead, and how earnestly I must exert myself in order to give in return as much as I have received.

Albert Einstein

We focused on self-care during the early weeks of recovery. It is fitting, near the end of one year, to reexamine the shifting balance of self-care and caregiving. As time and circumstances change, it is important to remain vigilant, continually assessing what you need for your own long-term recovery. *Self-care does not exclude caring for others.* But balance of care must be a consistent consideration for those who rarely care for themselves.

Ram Dass, stroke survivor and author of *Still Here,* expresses this caregiving paradox clearly: "We value taking care of others, but shun the notion of being taken care of ourselves. . . . Rather than opening our hands to accept what others have to offer, many of us close down. . . . Allowing ourselves to reveal our need, we allow those around us the opportunity to help, which is a fundamental need we all share."

Though more difficult when your partner has a serious illness, balancing self-care and caregiving is essential for your healing and well-being. Focus on giving and receiving, so that you are neither depleted nor concerned only for yourself.

Affirmation: I am learning to balance giving and receiving.

Related topics to think/write about:
1) My capacity to receive from others. 2) My needs that are being met at this period in my recovery, and those that are not.

Qualities to meditate on: Balance–individuality–receptivity.

196

Date _____

This is the _____ *week of my recovery* _____

_____
_____
_____
_____
_____
_____
_____
_____
_____
_____
_____
_____
_____
_____
_____
_____
_____
_____
_____
_____
_____
_____
_____
_____
_____
_____

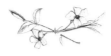

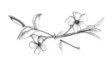

We'd always talked about buying a cabin and I'd completely ruled it out. I was afraid of being so far away. At a cabin in the woods, I wouldn't be close enough to an ambulance, a hospital, a doctor. What would happen if . . . ? We bought it! It was a celebration of my freedom to do things again without constantly worrying about the umbilical cord to the hospital.

Lavonne, a heartmate

Lavonne's story of celebration provides a snapshot of one moment in the lengthy mourning process. It illustrates a loss of dreams, a loss of freedom, a life dominated by fear and its accompanying limitations, and a new liberation.

The grief process includes expressing fear, changing priorities, acknowledging a new reality. But after many months, something changes in the bereaved. You wouldn't be a heartmate if you didn't sometimes feel fear. But having arrived at this new stage of recovery, you can begin to live again. When the fear comes, it is no longer more powerful than you are. It's less intense; it neither lasts as long nor paralyzes you.

Making your way through grief and fear, you once again find energy for and interest in the present and future. Though you may be unable to buy a second home or travel to a faraway place, each heartmate needs to mark this significant stage, the end of acute grief.

There is only now. You can choose to live today fully, joyously. Celebrate your new awareness together.

Affirmation: I freely celebrate life and living today.

Related topics to think/write about:
   1) How does fear still dominate my decisions and actions?
   2) How can I express more beauty, joy, love, and meaning in my life?

Qualities to meditate on: Liberation–strength–vitality.

200

Date _____

This is the ___ *week of my recovery* _____

_____

_____

_____

_____

_____

_____

_____

_____

_____

_____

_____

_____

_____

_____

_____

_____

_____

_____

_____

_____

_____

_____

_____

_____

_____

_____

_____

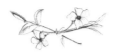

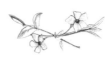

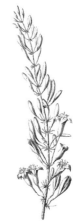

Each wound we suffer and eventually heal from is a soul-making experience with the potential to awaken our willingness to participate in the healing of the world.
Joan Borysenko
Fire in the Soul

In the early months, it's natural for heartmates, wounded by the health crisis, to experience depression and anger. As healing progresses and energy returns, many heartmates—and patients, too—want to help heal others.

Some express their gratitude by working with other families struggling with serious illness. Others participate in support groups for heartmates of cancer and AIDS survivors, where they listen and share their experience with those in similar situations. Still others have interests that take them far from illness, but the motivation is the same: to help heal our wounded planet. They serve the homeless, visit children in nurseries and shelters, mentor in literacy programs, work to save the environment.

There is no one right way to participate in healing. Joanna Macy writes in *Coming Back to Life,* "We are beginning to wake up, as from a millennia-long sleep, to a whole new relationship to our world, to ourselves and others." Healing presents an opportunity to search for a right and loving way to express what is in your heart.

Affirmation: In my unique way, I am a devoted citizen of this planet.

Related topics to think/write about:
1) My understanding of myself, having had "a soul-making experience."
2) My natural interests and concrete plans to act on them.

Qualities to meditate on: Dedication–healing–renewal.

204

Date _____

This is the _____ *week of my recovery* _____

_____

_____

_____

_____

_____

_____

_____

_____

_____

_____

_____

_____

_____

_____

_____

_____

_____

_____

_____

_____

_____

_____

_____

_____

_____

_____

_____

_____

_____

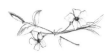

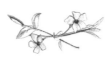

Let there be peace on earth and let it begin with me.
> Sy Miller and Jill Jackson,
> "Let There Be Peace on Earth"
> © Jan-Lee Music, 1955, 1983

No heartmate can take responsibility for the whole world, yet many feel guilty about not doing more when there is so much injustice, war, and poverty on earth. No single person can fix the world's ills, but each heartmate can work on inner peace and share it with the rest of us.

Although it's been almost a year since the journey with your mate's illness began, you're probably only beginning to experience peace with yourself. The drain on your energy has been significant. You've had losses to grieve. You and your family have had to learn a complex process: finding and accepting a new "normal" that includes a serious illness.

Most heartmates need at least one full calendar year to struggle with the feelings about what has happened. Even then, some heartmates still feel angry and confused about how to repair their relationship. Other heartmates are still learning about long-term lifestyle changes and how to think optimistically. Still others continue to cope with days of depression and disappointment.

Inner peace is a wonderful goal to work toward. Perhaps world peace can only come once we've each done the individual groundwork to find peace within ourselves.

Affirmation: Peace on earth, and let it begin with me.

Related topics to think/write about:
1) What peace looks like in my personal life, family life, and work life. 2) Paths I can take to inner peace in my everyday life.

Qualities to meditate on: Light–purpose–transformation.

208

Date _____

This is the   week of my recovery _____

_____

_____

_____

_____

_____

_____

_____

_____

_____

_____

_____

_____

_____

_____

_____

_____

_____

_____

_____

_____

_____

_____

_____

_____

_____

_____

_____

_____

_____

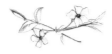

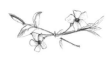

What we call the beginning is often the end
And to make an end is to make a beginning.
The end is where we start from.

T. S. Eliot

This is the fifty-second week in *The Heartmates Journal.* Happy anniversary and congratulations! You've completed a year of working on your recovery. You've reached the end of this book, but not the end of your healing journey.

It is important to acknowledge endings. "A new year can begin only because the old year ends," explains Madeleine L'Engle, author of the children's classic, *A Wrinkle in Time.* Endings and beginnings, turning points, anniversaries, family occasions, and achievements mark the special moments in life and prepare us to move forward.

Rituals can be delightful ways to observe endings. Heartmates' unique celebrations include planting a tree, creating a banner on your home computer, spending a romantic evening with your mate, and preparing and eating a special meal.

By now you are skilled at journaling as a method to reflect on your life, and at meditating to grow and capitalize on your strengths. If you'd like to continue using these techniques, you'll find additional quotations and qualities in the appendices of this book. Or you may want to wing it on your own now. One way to celebrate this end and beginning is to buy yourself a gift. How about a beautiful new journal to welcome the next period of your recovery?

Affirmation: I can say good-bye; I look forward to the next hello.

Related topics to think/write about:
1) Consider and plan celebrations to mark milestones in my life. 2) Things in my life that I now need to say good-bye to.

Qualities to meditate on: Celebration–delight–letting go.

Date _____

This is the _____ *week of my recovery* _____

_____
_____
_____
_____
_____
_____
_____
_____
_____
_____
_____
_____
_____
_____
_____
_____
_____
_____
_____
_____
_____
_____
_____
_____
_____
_____
_____
_____
_____
_____
_____
_____
_____

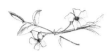

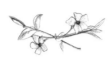

Appendix A: Recommended Reading List

This recommended reading list is divided by subject for your convenience. I have chosen books that are readable and practical to invite further exploration in areas that might be of interest to you.

On Illness, Caregiving, and Caregivers

At the Will of the Body: Reflections on Illness. Arthur W. Frank. Boston: Houghton Mifflin Company, 1991.

Finding Your Way: Families and the Cancer Experience: A Guidebook. Gail A. Noller, PsyD. Minneapolis: American Cancer Society, Minnesota Division, 1998.

Healing beyond Body: Medicine and the Infinite Reach of the Mind. Larry Dossey, MD. New York: Random House, 2001.

Healing Words: The Power of Prayer and the Practice of Medicine. Larry Dossey, MD. New York: Harper, 1997.

Heartmates: A Guide for the Spouse and Family of the Heart Patient. Third edition. Rachael Freed. Minneapolis: Fairview Press, 2002.

Helping Yourself Help Others: A Book for Caregivers. Rosalynn Carter, with Susan K. Golant. New York: Times Books, 1994.

Intimacy. Marilyn Mason, PhD, LCP. Center City, Minn.: Hazelden, 1986 (pamphlet).

Kitchen Table Wisdom. Rachel Naomi Remen, MD. New York: Riverhead Books, 1996.

Multiple Sclerosis: A Guide for Families. Rosalind C. Kalb, PhD. New York: Demos Vermande, 1998.

Still Here: Embracing Aging, Changing, and Dying. Ram Dass. New York: Penguin Putnam, 2000.

Transitions: Making Sense of Life's Changes. William Bridges. Reading, Mass.: Addison-Wesley, 1980.

Ways You Can Help: Creative, Practical Suggestions for Family and Friends of Patients and Caregivers. Margaret Cooke, with Elizabeth Putman. New York: Warner Books, 1996.

We Are Not Alone: Learning to Live with Chronic Illness. Sefra Kobrin Pitzele, New York: Workman Publishing, 1986.

On Grief and Loss

Companion through the Darkness: Inner Dialogues on Grief. Stephanie Ericsson.
    New York: HarperCollins, 1993.
Healing after Loss: Daily Meditations for Working through Grief. Martha Whitmore
    Hickman. New York: Avon Books, 1994.
Life after Loss: Conquering Grief and Finding Hope. Raymond Moody Jr., MD, and
    Dianne Arcangel. San Francisco: HarperSanFrancisco, 2001.
Necessary Losses. Judith Viorst. New York: Simon & Schuster, 1986.
Sailing. Susan Kenney. New York: Viking Penguin, 1988 (fiction).
Stones for Ibarra. Harriet Doerr. New York: Penguin Books, 1978 (fiction).
Two-Part Invention: The Story of a Marriage. Madeleine L'Engle. New York:
    Farrar, Straus & Giroux, 1988 (autobiography).
When Bad Things Happen to Good People. Rabbi Harold S. Kushner. New York:
    Schocken Books, 1981.

On Growth

Blessing: The Art and the Practice. David Spangler. New York: Riverhead
    Books, 2001.
Coming Back to Life: Practices to Reconnect Our Lives, Our World. Joanna Macy and
    Molly Young Brown. Gabriola Island, British Columbia: New Society
    Publishers, 1998.
Fire in the Soul: A New Psychology of Spiritual Optimism. Joan Borysenko, PhD.
    New York: Warner Books, 1993.
*Inevitable Grace: Breakthroughs in the Lives of Great Men and Women: Guides to
    Your Self-Realization.* Piero Ferrucci. Los Angeles: Jeremy P. Tarcher, 1990.
Lighting a Candle: Quotations on the Spiritual Life. Molly Young Brown, ed. New
    York: HarperCollins, 1994.
New Passages: Mapping Your Life across Time. Gail Sheehy. New York: Random
    House, 1995.
Soul Mates: Honoring the Mysteries of Love and Relationship. Thomas Moore. New
    York: HarperCollins, 1994.

On Healing

Forgive for Good. Frederic Luskin, PhD. New York: HarperCollins, 2001.
Healing into Immortality: A New Spiritual Medicine of Healing Stories and Imagery.
    Gerald Epstein, MD. New York: Bantam Books, 1994.

Healing Words: The Power of Prayer and the Practice of Medicine. Larry Dossey, MD. New York: HarperCollins, 1993.

Heart Illness and Intimacy: How Caring Relationships Aid Recovery. Wayne M. Sotile, PhD. Baltimore: The Johns Hopkins University Press, 1992.

Intentional Family: Simple Rituals to Strengthen Family Ties. William J. Doherty, PhD. New York: Avon, 1999.

Mainstay: For the Well Spouse of the Chronically Ill. Maggie Strong. Boston: Little, Brown, & Co., 1988.

The Power of the Mind to Heal. Joan Borysenko, PhD, and Miroslav Borysenko, PhD. Carson, Calif.: Hay House, 1994.

On Meditation

Healing into Life and Death. Stephen Levine. New York: Doubleday, 1987.

How to Meditate. Lawrence LeShan. New York: Bantam Books, 1974.

The Inner Guide Meditation. Edwin C. Steinbrecher. York Beach, Maine: Samuel Weiser, 1988.

On Writing and Journaling

The Artist's Way. Julia Cameron. New York: G. P. Putnam, 1992.

Ethical Wills: Putting Your Values on Paper. Barry K. Baines, MD. San Francisco: Perseus, 2002.

Life's Companion: Journal Writing as a Spiritual Quest. Christina Baldwin. New York: Bantam Books, 1990.

Women's Lives, Women's Legacies: Passing Your Beliefs and Blessings to Future Generations. Rachael Freed. Minneapolis: Fairview Press, 2003

On Mental Imagery and Ritual

The Art of Ritual: A Guide to Creating and Performing Your Own Rituals for Growth and Change. Renee Beck and Sydney Barbara Metrick. Berkeley: Celestial Arts, 1990.

Guided Meditations, Explorations and Healings. Stephen Levine. New York: Doubleday, 1991.

APPENDIX B: ADDITIONAL QUOTATIONS

Part I: Early Recovery

The myth is that everything will be the same as it was. The truth is that nothing will ever be the same again.

> Rachael Freed
> *Heartmates*

Being in a hospital at a time of serious illness is like living in a foreign country—you don't know the rules, you're always an outsider.

> David V. Keith, MD
> *Portrait of the Heartmate*

He's had to make substantial changes in his practice. So, layered with the other kinds of concerns is a real change of image, change in status, and a kind of acknowledged grieving.

> Ardis, a heartmate

My husband had to say good-bye forever to part of our life together. . . . He told me at the time that the most frustrating aspect of my illness was that he could not control what was happening. . . . We felt powerless for a long time after the diagnosis. . . . The more we talked, the more I came to understand that he had a very rich and complex picture of me as wife, lover, mother of his children, soul mate, partner, and friend. My illness was causing him to dismantle many of those pictures, one by one, against his will. He was grieving, too.

> Sefra Kobrin Pitzele
> *We Are Not Alone: Learning to Live with Chronic Illness*

There is nothing I can count on. I have to change my game plan. How can I hold on to myself and love her ? How do I integrate this into my life—give it the back bedroom, not the living room or the kitchen? I have very little tolerance for the superficial.

> Greg, a heartmate

Be patient with yourself. . . . When we lose something we love, often our ability to love life is also lost for a while.

> Noah ben Shea
> *Jacob's Journey: Wisdom to Find the Way, Strength to Carry On*

Much of the time I felt very much alone, except when I could pick up the telephone. . . .

> Gretchen, a heartmate

It is difficult for a caregiver to separate himself physically from the care receiver. Often, there is little or no opportunity to do so. Some caregivers feel guilty to admit it, but after a while, they feel trapped by their new responsibilities.

> Sefra Kobrin Pitzele
> *We Are Not Alone: Learning to Live with Chronic Illness*

Everything felt different. Living together was different; sleeping together was different.

> Ethelyn, a heartmate

It isn't easy to affirm your strengths. Most of us are more comfortable with criticism than with compliments. We find it difficult to appreciate our positive qualities, although we are acutely aware of our weaknesses. . . . [But] taking credit for doing your best is an important part of the recovery process.

> Rachael Freed
> *Heartmates*

It's normal to be angry . . . saddened. If you don't grieve over it, then you will carry it around as an invisible weight on your back . . . the same is true for the spouse!

> Robert Eliot, MD
> *Portrait of the Heartmate*

The impulse to protect your children from pain and anguish is universal. But the truth is that it's impossible to do. Even if you could protect your children from reality, it wouldn't necessarily be doing them a favor. Learning to cope with crisis . . . is a valuable part of growing up.

Rachael Freed
Heartmates

Support groups are crucial for your own well-being. [They] give you an opportunity to joke and laugh about your circumstances with people who really understand and won't judge you, [and they] give you an opportunity to cry and complain without others urging you to "buck up" or making you feel guilty about your own needs and pain.

Rosalynn Carter
Helping Yourself Help Others: A Book for Caregivers

We were probably all in a state of shock, because it was such an unexpected thing. On the other hand, there was something very calming, almost comforting about it, because we all knew that it wasn't in our hands at all.

Mary, a heartmate

Of all the care Cathie gave me, the most important was her willingness and ability to talk about what was happening to me, and to her. Through our talk illness did not happen just to me, it happened to us.

Arthur W. Frank, a heart and cancer patient
At the Will of the Body

A frequent problem is assuming that your partner knows what you need without [your] saying it. This is a new experience for both of you, and neither knows what the other needs unless you talk to each other.

Gail A. Noller, PsyD
Finding Your Way: Families and the Cancer Experience

What do you do? You're feeling emotional, afraid, vulnerable, and you're not the one with cancer. Keeping the lines of communication open will help you find ways to show affection to each other.

A heartmate
A Significant Journey: Breast Cancer Survivors and the Men Who Love Them (video)

Part II: Midrecovery

Making decisions that align your purpose with your values is difficult, particularly during the acute phase of a crisis, but also as you reorient your life during recovery. . . . Taking time to think about your decisions can keep you anchored to the values and purpose that are the foundation of your actions.

Rachael Freed
Heartmates

A deeper part of you knows that it's not going to go on forever. . . . The "shoulds" maybe aren't such a big deal anymore.

Ethelyn, a heartmate

First there is an ending, then a beginning, with an important empty or fallow time in between. . . . [It's a] three-phase process of ending, lostness, and beginning. . . . One of the first and most serious casualties . . . is our sense of and plans for the future.

William Bridges
Transition: Making Sense of Life's Changes

When we accommodate others without considering ourselves, the results can be harmful . . . giving other people our power to think and feel, putting another person in charge of us, while ignoring our own inner world of truth.

Marilyn Mason, PhD, LCP
Intimacy

Fear of the unknown can be fought only with faith and courage. You will never achieve peace of mind unless you come to terms with reality.

> Rachael Freed
> *Heartmates*

The fact was, I was totally dependent on him financially. I needed to change that in order to feel more secure in my life.

> Mary, a heartmate

Providing ways to help and support each other on our journeys to truth may be the highest form of love.

> Rob Lehman, a stroke survivor
> from *Still Here: Embracing Aging, Changing, and Dying*

If you don't take care of yourself, there will be nothing left for anyone else.

> Sefra Kobrin Pitzele
> *We Are Not Alone: Learning to Live with Chronic Illness*

When caregivers perceive themselves as being alone and in "second place" with no one to talk to or help out, they often feel trapped— literally imprisoned in their own households. These feelings can lead to intense anger and depression, which can further drive away friends and family.

> Rosalynn Carter
> *Helping Yourself Help Others: A Book for Caregivers*

I finally came to the conclusion that I couldn't live like this, because I was so concerned about his life. I developed the philosophy: in order to have life, I must live.

> Bonnie, a heartmate

Be generous in your expectations of yourself and your mate.

> Rachael Freed
> *Heartmates*

Be not without hope
For crystal rain falls from black clouds.
Persian poem

Part III: Toward Full Recovery

When the heart weeps for what it has lost,
The spirit laughs for what it has found.
Sufi aphorism

As serious and significant as your relationship is, nothing is a more powerful healer than humor. Being able to laugh at yourselves and your situation will help you see things as they truly are and enjoy your togetherness.
Rachael Freed
Heartmates

Coming close to death, having it almost in the room with us on several occasions, also makes us very aware of how beautiful our life is together and how many wonderful things we share.
Ardis, a heartmate

If the only prayer you say in your whole life is "thank you," that would suffice.
Meister Eckhart

The prairie has informed my life: wild, free, open, nonjudging, gentle and fierce. I just remember being wildly happy. I would get lost in the space between sky and earth. My memory of this gift seems to include no intellectual things, only glorious, intense, soul-sweet yearning to be connected to the prairie. Winter nights gave the gift of stars and northern lights. I know the prairie still runs in my blood and fuels every creative endeavor and is the place I feel at home on the earth.
From the journal of Kitty Kotchian Smith

One of the things you let go of in the ending process is the need to see the past in a particular way. . . . A new chapter of my life . . . is beginning. I haven't become somebody else.

William Bridges
Transitions: Making Sense of Life's Changes

It never occurred to me that he would ever get sick, that he wouldn't be there to be strong, pay the bills, help everybody who needed help, mow the lawn, fix the porch. And suddenly he was human. It made us equal. I feel closer to him and I think he feels closer to me, because I see him as he is and he's okay the way he is.

Lavonne, a heartmate

The caregiver often has more difficulty finding time and recognition for mourning. While I was ill we knew that she, the caregiver, needed to mourn and recognize losses as much as I, the ill person. We both had to let our grieving run its course.

Arthur W. Frank, a heart and cancer patient
At the Will of the Body

In resisting your grief, you deny yourself the good seeds born of grieving, seeds vital for planting a new crop of realistic dreams for the garden of your future. Trust yourself and the grief process. Your efforts will bear fruit.

Rachael Freed
Heartmates

Feeling needy and self-centered—cocooning—is a normal, instinctive act of self-protection during the acute period of crisis and the early stages of recovery. Your world got very tiny while you were preoccupied with your personal issues. . . . Recovery might be defined as the gradual process of moving back into relationship with the larger world around you. . . . As you emerge, like a chrysalis awaiting transformation to a butterfly, you may experience dissatisfaction, restlessness, and an urge to find new meaning in your life.

Rachael Freed
Heartmates

See our new circumstance as an opportunity for greater intimacy . . . the paradox of what we call misfortune: that so often what we most resist bestows on our lives the greatest, most unexpected blessings. . . . People who take care of someone who's dependent . . . come away feeling they've received a gift. And isn't that really the game of human relationships—that when we walk away, we both feel gifted from having been in the exchange?

> Ram Dass, a stroke survivor
> *Still Here: Embracing Aging, Changing, and Dying*

As much as you may yearn for the life before cancer, you can't return to the old normal. You and your family are forever changed. Your challenge is to create the new normal, finding a way to rebalance that family mobile. The way to begin is to grieve the losses and celebrate the gains. . . . Finally, there is resolution to the grief over loss. This is not "getting over it" but rather "getting used to it." It is a matter of integration, that is, making this experience of cancer a part of your life, your history, and your future.

> Gail A. Noller, PsyD
> *Finding Your Way: Families and the Cancer Experience*

Even though I take my responsibilities very seriously, I am not a martyr. I am the caregiver and perhaps I don't get out socially as much as I might want to, but I keep a part of me for just me. If I give all of me, I can be destroyed as an individual and then have nothing to give. I feel that everyone should have another interest that they are passionate about.

> Ruth, a heartmate

We don't stop playing because we grow old, we grow old because we stop playing.

> Anonymous

You have got to own your days and live them, each one of them, every one of them, or else the years go right by and none of them belong to you.

Herb Gardner
A Thousand Clowns

The task now is to find a new future self in whom we can invest our trust and enthusiasm.

Gail Sheehy
New Passages

We learn as much from sorrow as from joy, as much from illness as from health, from handicap as from advantage—and indeed perhaps more.

Pearl S. Buck

Grow old along with me!
The best is yet to be.

Robert Browning

APPENDIX C: AFFIRMATIONS

Affirmations from Part I: Early Recovery

I will be gentle and kind to myself today.
I will use my energy today to attend to what is truly important.
I accept the need to take care of myself.
I can change, a little bit every day.

I am entitled to have questions and answers.
I deserve support and I will ask for it.
I am strong; I will survive and thrive.
I have many strengths, including the ability to face reality
    and uncertainty.

I am capable of experiencing my grief and healing.
I do not stand alone; I am brave enough to reach out to my partner.
I protect my children best with my caring and honesty.
I accept the fact of uncertainty, the permanence of change.

My feelings are a normal response to the crisis I am experiencing.
I deserve to be touched in loving, respectful ways.
I am a worthwhile human being who can accommodate change.
I will express my love by stepping back and letting go.

I am strong enough to face my fears.
I am resilient; I can adapt to a life of uncertainty.
I am responsible for my own feelings, and no one else's.
I will do my part for our partnership.

Affirmations from Part II: Midrecovery

As my mate heals, I will use my power to relinquish control
    and any temporarily assumed roles.
I am human and in the hands of God or my higher power.
    I am being held by the universe.
I am learning to think realistically and optimistically.
I can master my fear by recognizing it and assessing real danger.

I can differentiate between being rightly responsible and
    being overresponsible.
I am loving, lovable, and desirable.
I trust my own pace.
I rejoice in the blessings of my life today.

I am more than what I do.
I am strong enough to experience my sadness and
    my disappointment.
I am entitled to experience the abundance of life.
I will respectfully acknowledge my feelings without judgment.

I will honor my grief by giving myself the time I need.
I will enjoy this moment.
My mate and I are separate, each of us individual and whole.
I will pay attention to what my mate's illness has to teach me.

I commit myself to the spiritual task of opening to the unknown.
I will love myself and my mate.
I will open myself to realistic trust.
I will use the energy of my anger constructively.

Affirmation from Part III: Toward Full Recovery

I am whole and a part of creation.
I celebrate the love and learning given me in my life as a parent.
I am strong enough to feel and master my fears.
I accept my strengths and my limitations.

I redefine myself as I integrate my worthiness.
I am preparing myself to live fully in the present by
    grieving past losses.
I will live as a blessing to myself and those around me.
I am learning to balance giving and receiving.

I freely celebrate life and living today.
In my unique way, I am a devoted citizen of this planet.
Peace on earth, and let it begin with me.
I can say good-bye; I look forward to the next hello.

APPENDIX D: QUALITIES

Qualities from Part I: Early Recovery

Week 1:   Calm–quiet–simplicity.
Week 2:   Order–rest–surrender.
Week 3:   Balance–energy–renewal.
Week 4:   Celebration–creativity–patience.

Week 5:   Appreciation–comprehension–humor.
Week 6:   Generosity–grace–openness.
Week 7:   Confidence–imagination–preparation.
Week 8:   Courage–perseverance–realism.

Week 9:   Strength–surrender–willingness.
Week 10:   Communication–intimacy–partnership.
Week 11:   Community–harmlessness–integrity.
Week 12:   Acceptance–serenity–wisdom.

Week 13:   Comprehension–faith–optimism.
Week 14:   Celebration–generosity–love.
Week 15:   Humor–power–resilience.
Week 16:   Cooperation–dedication–responsibility.

Week 17:   Liberation–power–understanding.
Week 18:   Determination–openness–truth.
Week 19:   Compassion–detachment–harmlessness.
Week 20:   Friendship–partnership–trust.

Qualities from Part II: Midrecovery

Week 21: Cooperation–creativity–responsibility.
Week 22: Letting go–surrender–trust.
Week 23: Control–enthusiasm–optimism.
Week 24: Calm–courage–humor.

Week 25: Freedom–goodwill–responsibility.
Week 26: Friendship–love–tenderness–trust.
Week 27: Balance–energy–realism.
Week 28: Acceptance–appreciation–gratitude.

Week 29: Comprehension–faith–wonder.
Week 30: Creativity–determination–flexibility.
Week 31: Abundance–adventure–play.
Week 32: Acceptance–detachment–serenity–understanding.

Week 33: Identity–integrity–meaning.
Week 34: Beauty–joy–light–play.
Week 35: Empowerment–responsibility–surrender.
Week 36: Compassion–meaning–partnership.

Week 37: Order–strength–universality.
Week 38: Generosity–harmony–peace.
Week 39: Clarity–faith–love–trust.
Week 40: Discernment–energy–vitality.

Qualities from Part III: Toward Full Recovery

Week 41:   Cooperation–harmony–wholeness.
Week 42:   Faith–gratitude–responsibility.
Week 43:   Courage–realism–serenity.
Week 44:   Acceptance–forgiveness–peace.

Week 45:   Authenticity–creativity–integrity.
Week 46:   Appreciation–humor–playfulness.
Week 47:   Compassion–education–service.
Week 48:   Balance–individuality–receptivity.

Week 49:   Liberation–strength–vitality.
Week 50:   Dedication–healing–renewal.
Week 51:   Light–purpose–transformation.
Week 52:   Celebration–delight–letting go.

LIST OF QUALITIES

abundance • acceptance • admiration • adventure
appreciation • awe • balance • beauty • being
belonging • bliss • brotherhood • celebration • change
clarity • communication • community • compassion
comprehension • control • cooperation • courage
creativity • dedication • delight • detachment
determination • ecstasy • education • efficiency
energy • enthusiasm • eternity • expectancy • faith
flexibility • forgiveness • freedom • friendship
generosity • goodness • goodwill • grace
gratitude • harmlessness • harmony • healing
honesty • humor • imagination • inclusiveness
individuality • inspiration • integration • integrity
intimacy • joy • letting go • liberation • love
loyalty • meaning • obedience • openness
optimism • order • partnership • patience • peace
perseverance • play • poise • positiveness • power
purification • purpose • quiet • realism • release
renewal • resilience • responsibility • rest
serenity • service • silence • simplicity • sisterhood
spontaneity • steadfastness • strength• surrender
synthesis • tenderness • transformation • trust
truth • understanding • unity • universality • vitality
wholeness • will • willingness • wisdom • wonder

APPENDIX E: IMAGERY TOOLS

The following imagery tools have been adapted from *Heartmates: A Guide for the Spouse and Family of the Heart Patient,* by Rachael Freed.

RELAXATION

Relaxing your body and mind is crucial to recovery. Biofeedback, yoga, and meditation are practical self-care practices that offer you a healthy way to manage the stress of a health crisis and revitalize yourself. Check local community education programs for available classes.

The following exercise is provided to get you started. It requires no more than ten minutes of your time. (Consider practicing it at the beginning or end of the day or whenever you take a break.) To maximize its effectiveness, do the exercise on a regular basis. Make it a priority in your daily routine.

You can practice this exercise on your own, with a friend, or with family members. Reading the exercise to yourself can be distracting, taking away from its effectiveness. Have someone else read the exercise to guide you (over time you will probably memorize the exercise). You can also record it. In either case, the reader should pause for a few seconds after each step, giving you time to follow the instructions.

Relaxation Exercise
Sit in a comfortable chair with your spine straight and your feet flat on the floor. Close your eyes and focus your attention on your breath. Follow its natural flow, in and out . . . in and out. . . . Take in clear, pure energy each time you inhale. Experience the release of tension as you exhale. . . . Don't change the pace of your breath in any way; your natural rhythm is perfect for you. Notice that with each breath you become more relaxed. . . .

Now focus on your body. Begin with your feet: first your right foot, then your left. Imagine all your tension flowing out through your toes and the bottoms of your feet. . . . Now allow the muscles in your calves and thighs to relax as well. First your right leg, now your left. Feel your legs warm and loose . . . feel how the muscles in your feet are relaxed. . . .

Now pay attention to your abdomen, where you may notice a distinct tightness. Let your breath fill your abdomen. . . . Exhale tension. . . . Now move your attention to your chest cavity, to where your heart is protected. Breathe in light to surround and fill your heart. . . . Feel the fullness, the freedom of release from worldly worries. . . .

Now focus on your back and your shoulders with their many muscles. Breathe energy into your back, your right shoulder, then your left. . . . Feel the tension loosen and slip from your body. . . . Feel your back and shoulders expand with the energy of the light. . . .

Now turn your focus to your arms and hands. First the right: Breathe pure energy into your upper arm, then the lower arm, and then into your hand. . . . Experience the tightness flowing out through your fingertips. . . . Now repeat, focusing on your left arm, hand, and fingers. . . .

Shift your focus to your neck and head. Feel your neck relax. . . . It gently holds your head above your body. Feel positive energy, the flow of light, run through it. . . . Concentrate now on your jaw, letting it relax, letting your mouth open naturally as you let go of holding it tight. . . . Now focus on your eyes; feel the muscles behind your eyes relaxing and expanding. . . . And last, be mindful of the top and back of your head. Feel your head get clear as the energy of light fills it. . . .

You are relaxed and alert. You are safe and present in this moment. You are filled with a sense of peace and well-being.

Now imagine yourself in a beautiful green meadow. . . . You are at rest, being nurtured by the beauty surrounding you. You are held securely by the solid earth beneath you. Feel the warm sun and the gentle cool breeze on your skin. . . . The air is fresh. You smell wildflowers and freshly mown grass. You hear birds singing to each other. A butterfly flutters by in the distance. You enjoy the babble of a nearby brook.

Let the peace and calm of this moment wash over you. . . . Allow yourself to soak in the feeling of safety . . . of being still. Stay in this serene and beautiful place as long as you like and are comfortable. . . . When you are ready, focus your attention on your breathing again. Breathe fully and deeply. . . . Breathe in a quality you can use when you return to your world—serenity . . . patience . . . freedom . . . compassion . . . forgiveness . . . love . . . and exhale any remaining tension or tightness. . . .

Now very gently bring yourself and your awareness back to the present and slowly open your eyes. . . . Take a moment to look around and return your awareness to the room . . . then rise slowly. . . . As you rise, stretch your body tall, fingertips reaching for the sky. . . . Now, with your sense of peace and your new quality, step into your reality refreshed and strengthened.

HEARTMATES® GUIDE FOR EXAMINING IMAGES

Purposeful examination of our images allows us to update them continually as time passes and conditions change. One of the advantages of taking stock and comparing past and present images is that you can appreciate new qualities you've developed in yourself as a response to your partner's illness.

- What do you recall about first visiting your mate in the hospital? In your mind's eye see your mate and the hospital unit as a still photo; then add sounds, smells, and movement to your image. What verbal and nonverbal messages did you receive from professional staff about your partner's condition? See yourself then. What were you feeling, thinking, doing? Describe your feelings and the quality of communication and intimacy with your mate.
- Create an image of your mate's physical illness. As much as you can, visualize the actual physical damage, as well as its symbolic meaning. How is your mate's physical and emotional body different since the onset of the disease? Now see the healing that

has occurred. Based on your image, how do you envision the long-term quality of your mate's life? Imagine yourself five, ten, and twenty years into the future. How has your mate's illness affected your lives? How do you expect this picture to change?

- What image of home and family do you have from the period of active recovery? What concerns did you have then about caring for your mate, your family, yourself? See in your mind's eye the network of communication and feelings that connected your family then. How was the family different during recovery from the way it was before the onset of the illness? What is your image of your family now? What issues are being dealt with now by your family? What is going well for all of you?

- Look into a mirror of your past. Who were you before your mate's health crisis? What was important to you? What was your relationship with your mate like? How was your daily life organized? What were your priorities? How did you define your purpose for living? Take this past image and set it aside.

- Stand in front of the same mirror right now. Who are you today? What do you know about your strengths and limitations? How do you feel about yourself now? What is important to you today? What is your relationship with your mate like? How do you organize your daily life? What are your priorities? What is your purpose for living? Take this present image and put it alongside your past image.

- Step back far enough so you can see both images in the mirror. Visualize how being a heartmate has changed you. What have you learned? How have you weathered the changes? In what ways have you taken responsibility for your recovery? How near or far are you from accepting what's happened to you? Have you forgiven yourself, your mate? Are you taking care of your most important needs? Which losses are you continuing to mourn? Which of your wounds have you healed and which need healing?

EVENING REVIEW

The Evening Review is an exercise particularly useful to people in a health crisis because it provides a structure to establish regular introspection, a quiet time when you can think about your day. "Re-viewing" can help you focus on vital questions raised by your partner's illness. Naturally operating during a crisis, "re-viewing" is a mental activity that helps to clarify reality, establish order in the midst of chaos, and structure a fresh perspective as you face uncertainty. The process of doing the exercise facilitates acceptance of reality in regular, small steps. The Evening Review, used daily, is a powerful recovery tool.

Evening Review Exercise

The Evening Review can be used to examine any particular aspect of your life, including inner processes or patterns you want to know more about. The exercise can be modified, too, to fit a specific need, as in the example on page 242, which applies to setting boundaries.

The attitude with which you approach your review is most important. When you examine your day, try to be a detached, objective observer, clearly registering what has happened without judgment or blame. Then move on to the next item of review without excitement, without elation at a success or disappointment about a failure. Aim for dispassionate awareness of your day. Don't relive it.

The review is best done as the last activity of your day. Before going to sleep, review your day going backward in time, "rewinding" it like a tape. Begin where you are right now, then observe evening, then the dinner hour, the afternoon, and so on backward through the morning to the moment you awoke.

Many people have found it valuable to write down observations, insights, or impressions in their journal. Doing so helps them process their thoughts, feelings, and perceptions. Taking notes or journaling is also a tool for remaining objective. It will help you "get out" of the subjectivity of your feelings, allowing you to discover patterns and trends in your thinking and perceiving. This becomes especially true if you review your notes over time.

Remember that the review is intended to be a mental tool. It is not for rehashing feelings or criticizing your decisions or actions. It is a tool for awareness, clarity, and understanding. It can lead to empowerment, healing, and change. Keep your review simple and defined. Give it no more than fifteen minutes a day (including any writing), particularly during the first weeks you practice it.

Review of Boundaries

The Evening Review can be applied to any aspect of your life that you want to see more clearly. The following modification consists of reviewing your day from the point of view of your boundaries. Boundaries are protective "membranes," personal lines of defense, best used to attract that which nourishes and sustains you and to deflect that which does not. (Consider the plant that soaks up nutrients in appropriate quantities.)

Before doing this review for the first time, identify activities and relationships that are particularly nourishing or depleting to you at this time in your life. Some additional things to keep in mind as a foundation for your Review of Boundaries, include:

- What is my experience of my boundaries? Have there been changes in my boundary system since the health crisis began? Are there changes as I become aware of my boundaries and how I use them?
- How do I evaluate environmental influences? Which give me comfort and which do I need protection from?
- How skillful am I in using and shifting my boundaries? In what situations and with which people is it easy or difficult to be me?
- What do I allow in? What do I push away? What in myself do I protect (my heart, my mind, my body, my feelings)?

You may consider these questions during the review itself, or you can consider them at the end of your review. They are meant to stimulate your thinking, to increase awareness about your boundaries and your needs as you heal from a crisis. After a week or two of doing the boundary review, take time to revisit your notes, looking for patterns and trends. You can use what you learn from your reviews to make decisions about setting firmer boundaries where necessary and relaxing or modifying those that are too restrictive.

Focus on moving through your day, doing a short overview from the present moment back to when you awoke for the day. Divide the periods of the day by your activities. First take a mental snapshot of your evening. If you notice anything about boundaries, jot them down in your journal. Next look at the dinner hour. Ask yourself to notice your boundaries in relation to those with whom you prepared or ate dinner. Continue to go backward from the afternoon to the morning, focusing on how your boundaries did or did not protect you during each activity.

When you are finished, set your journal aside. Do this for a minimum of a week before you reread your notes or try to distinguish a tendency or pattern.

PARTIAL LIFE REVIEW

People move through dark times into the light as they search for meaning. One of the natural ways people search is by reviewing what has happened to them in a crisis. This review is designed to help you analyze a transition or loss that you experienced *prior* to your mate's illness.

The exercise is particularly useful for identifying strengths as well as other qualities developed in past crises that you can apply and rely on now. Observe how you've handled loss in the past. Familiarize yourself with your unique patterns of coping. Your coping skills will expand as you see your strengths. You can incorporate the best of what you've done in the past with your newly developed skills and understanding.

You may want to do this review more than once, focusing on other life transitions. When you are familiar with your coping process, use the exercise to look at your present health crisis. Keep writing materials nearby. Insights, like dreams, are quickly forgotten unless they are recorded.

Partial Life Review Exercise

Take a few minutes to reflect on several events that were turning points in your life. Begin by jotting them down on paper. They might include a major decision you made, the loss of a relationship, or something that happened in society or in nature that had an impact on your life.

Now, from those events you have written down, choose one that you are willing to look at in a more detailed way. Recall the period of your life when the event happened. What was going on within you, outside you? Who were the important people in your life? Did you confide in anyone? Were you alone, without support? As you review this period of your life, see yourself as you were then.

Now recall how you acted, what kinds of things you did when the event first occurred. Did you respond differently after the first few weeks? If you did, how so?

Notice your feelings about what was happening to you. Was there a progression of feelings as time passed, as you integrated the experience into your life? Did you express your feelings directly, or did you keep them to yourself and try to forget them? Did you express some feelings and suppress others? Did your feelings come out indirectly? Did anyone important to you know how you were feeling?

Now recall your thoughts at the time of the event. What were you aware of, considering, weighing, judging? Did you do that thinking alone or was there someone with whom you discussed those thoughts? At the time, did you ever think that what was happening was an opportunity? Did it make sense to you personally? How about in the larger context of your life, the life of your family, community?

Now, come back to the present, aware that the event was *then* and this is *now*. Does the event make sense in relation to your life now? Is there something you can see about it now that you couldn't see then? Does this review change in any way how you see yourself? Are you now more understanding, compassionate, accepting, and forgiving of what you did, how you felt, or what you thought of yourself then? Is there anything you learned then (a skill or a quality that you developed) that you can use now?

Is there anything in this review that points toward your future, any new way you'd like to act, live, think, or feel? Are there positive implications for the future, now that you have reviewed the past in this structured way?

When you have finished your review, take time to write about what you've learned. If it makes sense to continue the process, you may want to share your review with someone important in your life. You may want to continue your observation of this event, its implications, or the patterns revealed. Use the Evening Review for that purpose.

BIBLIOGRAPHY

Assagioli, Roberto. *The Act of Will.* New York: Viking Press, 1973.

_____. *Psychosynthesis: A Manual of Principles and Techniques.* New York: Penguin Books, 1965.

Bolen, Jean Shinoda, MD. *The Tao of Psychology, Synchronicity and the Self.* San Francisco: Harper & Row, 1979.

Borysenko, Joan, PhD. *Fire in the Soul: A New Psychology of Spiritual Optimism.* New York: Warner Books, 1993.

Borysenko, Joan, PhD, and Miroslav Borysenko, PhD. *The Power of the Mind to Heal.* Carson, Calif.: Hay House, 1994.

Boss, Pauline. *Ambiguous Loss: Learning to Live with Unresolved Grief.* Cambridge, Mass.: Harvard University Press, 1999.

Bowman, Ted, MSW. *Loss of Dreams: A Special Kind of Grief.* (2111 Knapp Street, St. Paul, Minnesota 55108; phone or fax: 651-645-6058.)

Bridges, William. *Transitions: Making Sense of Life's Changes.* Reading, Mass.: Addison-Wesley Publishing, 1980.

Brown, Molly Young, ed. *Lighting a Candle: Quotations on the Spiritual Life.* New York: HarperCollins, 1994.

Cameron, Julia. *The Artist's Way: A Spiritual Path to Higher Creativity.* New York: Tarcher, 1992.

Carter, Rosalynn, with Susan K. Golant. *Helping Yourself Help Others: A Book for Caregivers.* New York: Times Books, 1994.

Cousins, Norman. *The Healing Heart.* New York: W. W. Norton, 1983.

Dass, Ram. *Still Here: Embracing Aging, Changing, and Dying.* New York: Penguin Putnam, 2000.

Doherty, William J., PhD. *Intentional Family: Simple Rituals to Strengthen Family Ties.* New York: Avon, 1999.

Dossey, Larry, MD. *Healing beyond Body: Medicine and the Infinite Reach of the Mind.* New York: Random House, 2001.

_____. *Healing Words: The Power of Prayer and the Practice of Medicine.* New York, Harper, 1997.

Ferrucci, Piero. *Inevitable Grace: Breakthroughs in the Lives of Great Men and Women: Guides to Your Self-Realization.* Los Angeles: Jeremy P. Tarcher, 1990.

Fowler, James W. *Stages of Faith.* San Francisco: Harper & Row, 1981.

Frank, Arthur W. *At the Will of the Body: Reflections on Illness.* Boston: Houghton Mifflin Company, 1991.

Freed, Rachael. *Heartmates: A Guide for the Spouse and Family of the Heart Patient.* Minneapolis: Fairview Press, 2002.

Herman, Judith, MD. *Trauma and Recovery.* New York: Basic Books, 1997.

Jackson, Jill, and Sy Miller. "Let There Be Peace on Earth." Occidental, Calif.: Jan-Lee Music, 1955, 1983.

Kabat-Zinn, Jon. *Full Catastrophe Living: Using the Wisdom of Your Body and Mind to Face Stress, Pain, and Illness.* New York: Dell, 1990.

Kalb, Rosalind C., PhD. *Multiple Sclerosis: A Guide for Families.* New York: Demos Vermande, 1998.

Kübler-Ross, Elisabeth, MD. *On Death and Dying.* New York: Macmillan, 1969.

Kushner, Harold S. *When All You've Ever Wanted Isn't Enough: The Search for a Life That Matters.* New York: Simon & Schuster, 1986.

_____. *When Bad Things Happen to Good People.* New York: Schocken Books, 1981.

Levin, Rhoda F. "Life Review: A Natural Process." *Readings in Psychosynthesis: Theory, Process, and Practice.* Toronto: Ontario Institute for Studies in Education, 1985.

Luskin, Frederic, PhD. *Forgive for Good.* New York: HarperCollins, 2001.

Macy, Joanna, and Molly Young Brown. *Coming Back to Life: Practices to Reconnect Our Lives, Our World.* Gabriola Island, British Columbia: New Society Publishers, 1998.

Maslow, Abraham H. *The Farther Reaches of Human Nature.* New York: Penguin Books, 1971.

Moody, Raymond Jr., MD, and Dianne Arcangel. *Life after Loss: Conquering Grief and Finding Hope.* San Francisco: HarperSanFrancisco, 2001.

Moore, Thomas. *Soul Mates: Honoring the Mysteries of Love and Relationship.* New York: HarperCollins, 1994.

Noller, Gail A., PsyD. *Finding Your Way: Families and the Cancer Experience: A Guidebook.* Minneapolis: American Cancer Society, Minnesota Division, 1998.

Northrup, Christiane, MD. *Women's Bodies, Women's Wisdom: Creating Physical and Emotional Health and Healing.* New York: Bantam Books, 1994.

Ornish, Dean, MD. *Love and Survival: The Scientific Basis for the Healing Power of Intimacy.* New York: HarperCollins, 1998.

Pitzele, Sefra Kobrin. *We Are Not Alone: Learning to Live with Chronic Illness.* New York: Workman Publishing, 1986.

Remen, Rachel Naomi, MD. *Kitchen Table Wisdom.* New York: Riverhead Books, 1996.

_____. *My Grandfather's Blessings.* New York: Riverhead Books, 2000.

Scarf, Maggie. *Intimate Partners: Patterns in Love and Marriage.* New York: Random House, 1987.

_____. *Intimate Worlds: Life inside the Family.* New York: Random House, 1995.

Scott-Maxwell, Florida. *The Measure of My Days.* New York: Penguin Books, 1979.

Seligman, Martin E. P., PhD. *Learned Optimism.* New York: Alfred A. Knopf, 1990.

Sheehy, Gail. *New Passages: Mapping Your Life across Time.* New York: Random House, 1995.

Siegal, Diana Laskin, et al. *The New Growing Older: Women Aging with Knowledge and Power.* New York: Touchstone Books, 1994.

Smedes, Lewis B. *The Art of Forgiving: When You Need to Forgive and Don't Know How.* New York: Ballantine Books, 1997.

Sotile, Wayne M., PhD. *Heart Illness and Intimacy: How Caring Relationships Aid Recovery.* Baltimore: The Johns Hopkins University Press, 1992.

Spangler, David. *Blessing: The Art and the Practice.* New York: Riverhead Books, 2001.

Strong, Maggie. *Mainstay: For the Well Spouse of the Chronically Ill.* Boston: Little, Brown, & Co., 1988.

Viorst, Judith. *Necessary Losses.* New York: Simon & Schuster, 1986.

Important Phone Numbers:

Emergency   911
Family Doctor
Specialist
Specialist
Specialist
Hospital
Favorite Nurse
Clergy
Pharmacy
Other

Prescriptions:

Drug Name
Prescription Number
Dosage
Side Effects

Drug Name
Prescription Number
Dosage
Side Effects

Drug Name
Prescription Number
Dosage
Side Effects

Drug Name
Prescription Number
Dosage
Side Effects

Doctor/Rehab Appointments:

Date/Time _____ Dr. _____

Date/Time _____ Dr. _____

Date/Time _____ Dr. _____

Date/Time _____ Dr. _____

Date/Time _____ Dr. _____

Date/Time _____ Dr. _____

Date/Time _____ Dr. _____

Date/Time _____ Dr. _____

Date/Time _____ Dr. _____

Questions (for the doctor, hospital personnel, clergy, etc.):

Notes:

Notes:

Notes:

Notes:

ABOUT THE AUTHOR

Rachael Freed, LICSW, LMFT, is a pioneer in family-centered care and the creator of the Heartmates resources, including *Heartmates: A Guide for the Spouse and Family of the Heart Patient* and *The Heartmates Journal: A Companion for Partners of People with Serious Illness*. Known internationally as an inspirational speaker, Rachael offers seminars for healthcare professionals and programs for cardiac couples. To inquire about a speaking engagement or workshop, email rachaelfreed@heartmates.com, or write to:

> Rachael Freed
> c/o Heartmates
> P.O. Box 16202
> Minneapolis, MN 55416

Rachael is also cofounder of The Legacy Center, which assists individuals in creating their spiritual-ethical will, and is the author of *Women's Lives, Women's Legacies: Passing Your Beliefs and Blessings to Future Generations*. She has five grandchildren: Sophie and Sam Stillman, and Mitch, Lily, and Harry Levin. Rachael lives in Minneapolis.